feelgood food

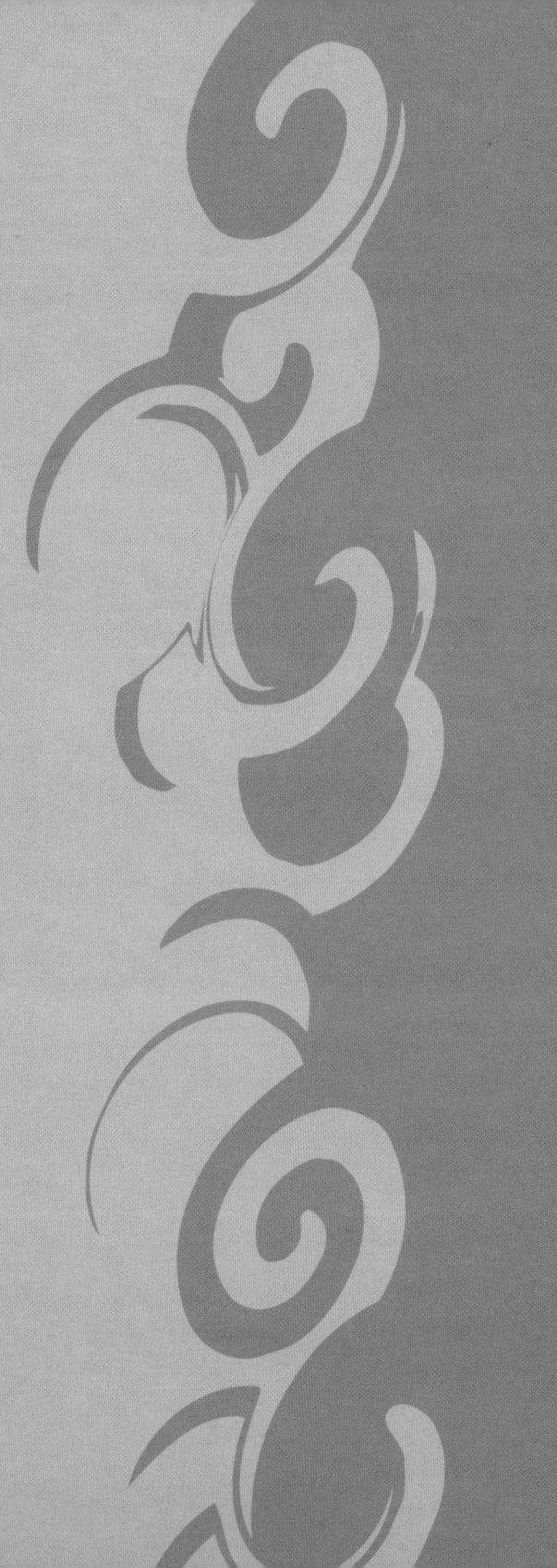

feelgood food

Recipes & menus for healthier Australian families

Mim Beim
&
Gül McCarty

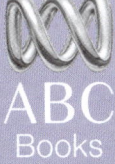
ABC Books

contents

ABOUT THE AUTHORS 7
INTRODUCTION 9
EATING PLANS 11

Acne 13
Anaemia 14
Arthritis 15
Asthma & coughing 16
Cancer prevention 17
Candida 18
Circulation 19
Colds 20
Cold sores 21
Constipation 22
Cystitis 23
Diabetes NIDDM 24
Diarrhoea 25
Eczema 26
Eye health 27
Gluten intolerance 28
Gum disease 29
Hayfever & sinus 30
Headache 31
Heart disease 32
Immune system 33
Inflammatory bowel disease 34

Insomnia	35
Irritable bowel syndrome	36
Lactose intolerance	37
Menopause & osteoporosis	38
Mouth ulcers	39
Nausea, morning sickness & travel sickness	40
Overweight	41
PMS & period problems	42
Prostate	43
Psoriasis	44
Stress	45
Tonsillitis & sore throat	46
THE RECIPES	48
Breakfast	51
Lunch	71
Lunchboxes	95
Dinner	107
Treats	139
Snacks	157
Drinks	171
MENU PLANS	187
YOUR PANTRY	191
DETOX … IF YOU MUST	196
YOUR FOOD JOURNAL	198
DON'T FORGET THE OTHER MEMBERS OF YOUR FAMILY	207

About the authors

Mim Beim

With over 18 years' experience as a naturopath, Mim Beim has developed a down-to-earth approach to healing. She believes that eating well is one of the fundamentals of good health and that a good diet should be a pleasure rather than a tortuous restriction of food. The author of five other books on natural therapies, Mim has also hosted two TV series on Foxtel's Lifestyle channel. She's a regular columnist for magazines and newspapers, and frequently broadcasts on ABC Radio. Mim currently holds the position of Head of Naturopathy for the ATMS, Australia's largest natural therapies association.

Gül McCarty

Gül has a varied background. Before turning her attention to health, fitness and writing, she was involved for many years in the food, finance, property development and real estate industries.

When she became ill with chronic fatigue in the 1980s, Gül started to make changes to her lifestyle, taking particular interest in nutrition. In the 1990s, to help out her sister, a working mother with a young son, she started cooking family meals. This led her to starting Kids' Kitchen, a business that supplied fresh healthy foods to day-care centres, feeding up to 500 children a day. Kids' Kitchen also specialised in catering for children with food allergies and other special needs. Later, the business expanded into manufacturing prepackaged meals for school canteens. Gül owned and managed commercial kitchen operations for over a decade.

Gül's Turkish background flavours many of her recipes, which incorporate traditional herbs and simple wholesome foods with fresh ingredients. She is passionate about good food and good health.

Introduction

Food plays a huge role in our daily lives. Among other things, we use it as fuel for our bodies; for its medicinal properties; for comfort; as a reward; as a gift; and for entertainment. But many of us see food preparation as just another dull, time-consuming chore, especially those trying to juggle families and jobs, financial commitments, health and fitness, medical conditions and so on. If 6pm comes around and you still haven't decided what's for dinner, then you've left your run too late. In the absence of forward planning and basic nutritional nous, slowly but surely, inappropriate food choices—in the form of a hamburger or fish and chips from the local takeaway—start to creep into our diet and our nutritional requirements go by the wayside. In no time, the kilos pile on, lethargy sets in, and the distinction between good and bad food becomes a blur.

Eating a variety of foods is important for your family's good health, but try telling that to a fastidious toddler or teenager. As tempting as it is to choose takeaway over a tantrum, letting children dictate what they will and won't eat is a flawed strategy—be fair but firm. In their defence, children can't be expected to understand what defines a well-balanced meal, so it falls to parents to educate them. Set good examples by eating well yourself; one of the best and easiest ways to do this is to, where possible, eat the same thing as your children. This is why *Feelgood Food* is such a gem. All the healthy and practical recipes that follow are suitable for every family member (except babies under one). This book proves unequivocally that healthy food can indeed be delicious. Rest assured, years of eating well-planned, tasty meals will eventually rub off on your children—and they might even thank you for your foresight down the track.

While not conceived as a book for sick people, *Feelgood Food* offers an abundance of foods that treat—and prevent—a range of medical conditions, from acne to cystitis to tonsillitis. We prefer you to use fresh, seasonal foods, so if you like the recipe, and the foods are affordable and in season, incorporate them into your weekly diet until the season ends.

If you're stumped for interesting meal ideas, our easy-to-follow menu plans will set you on the right path morning, noon and night. Once you get used to thinking about the daily nutritional needs of your family and plan accordingly, food preparation will become a breeze—even enjoyable—and mealtimes surprisingly stress-free. And once you've got a clear idea about which foods to seek out and which to avoid—and what food combinations work for you—by all means look beyond *Feelgood Food*. Look through the cookbooks on your shelf and your recipe clipping files for food ideas that you know will work for you and your family.

We wanted to share our passion for good food and good health with you and encourage you to think twice about what you put in your mouth. We hope we've achieved that. May you be unstoppable in your quest for a healthier and happier life.

Mim and Gül

Eating plans

food & recipes for common and chronic health complaints

The following pages contain eating plans to help manage a range of the most common and chronic health complaints that you may confront when preparing meals for your family and friends. Here are some tips on how to make the most of our suggestions and recommendations:

- The italicised recipes contain the key ingredients specifically recommended for this condition. Eat these meals at least four times a week or daily, if practical. Of course, if the recipe contains food you dislike, find a substitute—enjoying your food is as much a part of good health as the food itself. There are many roads to good health, and there will no doubt be another food or supplement that will be just as beneficial.

- Yoghurt: use plain whole milk, cow, sheep, goat or water buffalo made with acidophilus, bifidus cultures.

- What to eat: Enjoy a few or all 3–4 (or more) times a week.

- What to avoid: Try to avoid completely or have just once a week.

- Trigger foods. A number of conditions—for example, eczema, asthma and arthritis—may be triggered by food allergies/sensitivities. Not all people with a certain condition will have a problem with the same foods. If you aren't sensitive to a food, then it won't be harmful for your condition. For this reason, if you want to know if a trigger food poses a problem for you, eliminate it completely from your diet for one month. If there is no positive change in your condition, then it is unlikely that the food is a concern for you, and so it can be eaten freely.

- If a recipe calls for a minor ingredient appearing on the list of what to avoid, then enjoy the meal without that ingredient.

- Juicing is an excellent way to boost your quota of therapeutic nutrients. Vegetables and herbs, including carrots, beetroot, celery and parsley, make great juicing companions. And fruits such as berries, bananas and apricots go well in smoothies. Each eating plan features juice suggestions for your health condition.

- The recommended foods are a combination of traditional naturopathic remedies and foods that include substances that have proven beneficial in the treatment of certain conditions. For example, glucosamine is helpful in the treatment and prevention of arthritis, and is found in oats, oysters, tripe and okra. Indoles, which are found in broccoli and the rest of the Cruciferous family, are believed to help prevent some cancers.

- Wherever possible, buy and eat organic food. Organic food has been produced without the use of artificial pesticides, herbicides, fertilisers, fungicides and veterinary drugs (antibiotics, growth hormones), and the animals are often farmed more humanely. Although organic food is usually more expensive, it is better for our health and the environment. However, if organics are not available, or are outside your budget, then eat the freshest produce you can find.

- If reducing milk products, then make sure you eat plenty of calcium-rich foods.

- Food as medicine: The recipes that follow contain foods that may help in the treatment or prevention of various conditions and illnesses. Food is more than just fuel for the body. Certain foods can be therapeutic as well as nutritious—for example, yoghurt contains good bacteria (probiotics) that may help restore intestinal balance after antibiotics, as well as treat and prevent candida, cystitis and diarrhoea and help prevent certain types of bowel cancer.

- Allergies: Food allergies are becoming more common in Australia, particularly among children. 'Food allergies' is a catch-all phrase used to describe a wide variety of reactions to foods. This imprecision stems from the fact that food allergies is a relatively new area of accepted nutritional research. A true food allergy involves the body's immune system. After digestion a particular substance in a food alerts the immune system and an allergic reaction results, ranging from severe (for example, an anaphalyctic response to peanuts or shellfish) or to non-life threatening, such as wheezing, eczema, abdominal discomfort or hayfever. Food sensitivities are more subtle and symptoms may not show themselves for several days after eating a particular food. A food intolerance is where the body is unable to process the food substance—for instance, lactose in milk products or gluten in grains, including wheat.

Acne

What to eat

Fish, whole grains, legumes, nuts, all seeds (especially pepitas), seafood (especially oysters), parsley, garlic, sweet potato and apricots.

What to avoid

Sugar, milk products, especially yellow cheese, margarine and deep-fried foods.

Home help

Water is your skin's best friend. Drink 2–3 litres daily. You will also notice a big difference in your complexion if you drink the Vegetable cocktail every day.

Even though your skin may feel oily, it's important to keep moisturising. A blocked oil (sebum) gland is the nasty bit of the pimple. If skin is squeaky dry, oil glands will pump harder, causing more problems. Use a tea-tree-oil-based cleanser and moisturiser.

Menu choices

These recipes offer a combination of ideal foods for acne.

Breakfast
Toasted muesli with yoghurt
Mango, banana & tofu smoothie
Fruit salad with mint & yoghurt
Poached eggs with spinach & yoghurt

Lunch
Tuna salad
Mediterranean salad
Lentil salad
Minestrone with pesto
Brown rice & tuna salad
Carrot & ginger soup with coriander

Dinner
Marlin with green beans, pesto & roast tomatoes
Almost shepherd's pie (no cheese)
Garlic prawns
Mediterranean fish soup
Lentil stew

Snack
Chickpea & tahini dip
Beetroot & yoghurt dip

Treat
Mixed berries in blackcurrant jelly (no cream)
Pumpkin pudding with nutmeg & walnuts
Apricot & tofu pudding
Stewed apricots with honey yoghurt & almonds
Pumpkin & pepita muffins
Oat & sunflower-seed cookies

Drink
Iced spiced green tea
Vegetable cocktail (daily)

Juice companions

Try carrot, celery or beetroot added to your favourite base juice. Sip lemon juice, mixed with hot water, in the mornings. Avoid the sweeter fruit juices, which are high in sugar.

Anaemia

What to eat

Lamb, beef, chicken, fish (especially salmon and tuna), dried fruit (especially apricots, raisins, dates, figs and prunes), eggs, molasses, parsley, walnuts, leafy green vegetables (spinach, Chinese greens), leeks, lentils, kidney beans, sesame seeds, tofu, pumpkin, watercress, cherries, mulberries, strawberries, raspberries, broccoli and cocoa (also see Iron p115).

What to avoid

Tea or coffee drunk with or within half an hour of a meal.

Home help

Vitamin C increases iron absorption, so squeeze lemon juice over meals with meat or iron-rich vegetables. If this isn't appropriate, drink a glass of orange, tomato, guava or cranberry juice with meals that contain iron-rich foods.

Menu choices

These recipes offer a combination of ideal foods for anaemia.

Breakfast
Toasted muesli with yoghurt
Baked brown rice pudding
Poached eggs with spinach & yoghurt
Eggs with tomato, feta & herbs
Omelette with feta & dill

Lunch
All meals with beef, lamb or veal
Lentil salad

Dinner
All meals with beef, lamb or veal
Honey & soy chicken with rice
Lentil stew
Mediterranean fish soup

Snack
Beetroot & yoghurt dip

Treat
Chocolate polenta cake with choc chips
Apricot & tofu pudding
Stewed apricots with honey yoghurt & almonds
Oat & sunflower-seed cookies
Chocolate & raspberry muffins

Drink
Hot cocoa
Vegetable cocktail

Juice companions

Try all berries, apricots, spinach, beetroot, parsley, orange or lemon added to your favourite base juice.

Arthritis—osteo & rheumatoid

What to eat

Fish, green-lipped mussels, okra, cherries, green tea, cinnamon, pineapple, blueberries, blackberries, garlic, onions, Brussels sprouts, cabbage, broccoli, ginger, tripe, oats, oysters, alfalfa, carrot, avocados, nuts, seeds and olive oil.

What to avoid

Red meat, white flour products, sugar. Trigger foods may include oranges, tomato, capsicum, eggplant, potato, and tobacco.

Home help

An old-fashioned Vermont remedy says to add 1 teaspoon of apple cider vinegar with raw honey to 1 cup of hot water and drink it first thing each morning.

Menu choices

These recipes offer a combination of ideal foods for osteo and rheumatoid arthritis.

Breakfast

Toasted muesli with yoghurt
Mango, banana & tofu smoothie
Fruit salad with mint & yoghurt
Sardines & tomato on toast

Lunch

Tuna salad
Minestrone with pesto
Brown rice & tuna salad (no peanuts)
Carrot & ginger soup with coriander

Dinner

Marlin with green beans, pesto & roast tomatoes
Chickpea curry
Mediterranean fish soup

Snack

Spicy avocado mash on garlic toast

Treat

Mixed berries in blackcurrant jelly
Pumpkin pudding with nutmeg & walnuts
Apricot & tofu pudding
Stewed apricots with honey yoghurt & almonds
Pumpkin & pepita muffins
Oat & sunflower-seed cookies

Drink

Iced spiced green tea
Pear & ginger juice
Vegetable cocktail

Juice companions

Try pineapple, berries, ginger, carrot or celery added to your favourite base juice.

Asthma & coughing

What to eat

Garlic, onions, carrots, apricots (fresh and non-sulphur dried), walnuts, ginger, pumpkin, almonds, fish, avocados, olive oil, ginger, thyme, sweet potato and cloves.

What to avoid

Salt. Trigger foods may include shellfish, peanuts, milk products, chocolate, oranges, fruit bars, soft drinks, sausages, deli meats and food additives.

Home help

Slice 1 red onion, spread each slice with raw runny honey, place on a saucer and press the slices back together. Leave for 8 hours in a warm place. Take 2 teaspoons of the resulting fluid 3 times a day. This is good for any cough, including asthmatic coughing.

Also, a strong cup of black tea can help open the airways.

Menu choices

These recipes offer a combination of ideal foods for asthma and coughing.

Breakfast
Mango, banana & tofu smoothie
Fruit salad with mint & yoghurt
Sardines & tomato on toast

Lunch
Mediterranean salad
Beef salad
Spanish omelette with feta & dill
Minestrone with pesto
Brown rice & tuna salad
Red lentil soup
Carrot & ginger soup with coriander

Dinner
Honey & soy chicken with rice
Moroccan lamb with couscous
Marlin with green beans, pesto & roast tomatoes
Roast lamb with root vegetables
Roast beef with mustard, chives & garlic
Almost shepherd's pie (no cheese)
Chilli con carne with avocado & yoghurt topping
Chickpea curry
Garlic prawns
Mediterranean fish soup

Snack
Eggplant & tahini dip
Chickpea & tahini dip
Spicy avocado mash on garlic toast

Treat
Mixed berries in blackcurrant jelly (no cream)
Apple & walnut pie
Pumpkin pudding with nutmeg & walnuts
Stewed apricots with honey yoghurt & almonds
Apricot & tofu pudding

Drink
Iced lemongrass tea
Lemonade with mint leaves
Pear & ginger juice
Peppermint tea
Carrot, apple & orange juice
Vegetable cocktail

Juice companions

Try lemon, pineapple, ginger or carrot added to your favourite base juice.

Cancer prevention

What to eat

Soy, all sprouts, almonds, berries, spinach, watercress, sweet potato, nuts, shiitake mushrooms, carrots, apples, quinces and pears (eat seeds and all), linseeds, raw fruit and vegetables, green tea, seaweed, parsley, coriander; zucchini, green beans, cabbage, broccoli and beetroot. All antioxidant foods (see p183).

What to avoid

Sugar, white flour products, additives, excess alcohol, fried or fatty foods, deli meats and reduce red meat.

Home help

The cause of cancer remains unknown, though genetics, environmental toxins and stress are all believed to play a part. Diet has an important role to play in prevention. While a super-strict diet is counterproductive, ensure you eat plenty of fruit and vegetables, legumes and nuts, because they are high in antioxidants. Reducing stress is very important.

Menu choices

These recipes offer a combination of ideal foods for cancer prevention.

Breakfast
Toasted muesli with yoghurt
Mango, banana & tofu smoothie
Fruit salad with mint & yoghurt
Poached eggs with spinach & yoghurt

Lunch
Tuna salad
Lentil salad
Spanish omelette with feta & dill
Minestrone with pesto
Red lentil soup
Carrot & ginger soup with coriander

Dinner
Chickpea curry
Great northern beans
Lentil stew

Snack
Beetroot & yoghurt dip
Chickpea & tahini dip
Spicy avocado mash on garlic toast

Treat
Mixed berries in blackcurrant jelly (no cream)
Pumpkin pudding with nutmeg & walnuts
Apricot & tofu pudding
Stewed apricots with honey yoghurt & almonds
Pumpkin & pepita muffins
Oat & sunflower-seed cookies

Drink
Carrot, apple & orange juice
Iced spiced green tea
Vegetable cocktail
Peppermint tea with ginger

Juice companions

Try berries (all fruit, but not too sweet), parsley, spinach, celery, carrot or cabbage added to your favourite base juice.

Candida (thrush)

What to eat

Garlic, yoghurt, legumes, fish, chicken, meat, vegetables, fruit (except grapes, melons and dried fruits), miso and coconut.

What to avoid

Sugar, dried fruits, yellow and blue cheese, beer, wine, yeasted bread, fruit juice, grapes, melons and mushrooms.

Home help

To beat yeast infections, stick to a strict no-yeast, no-sugar diet for 6 weeks and eat 2–3 cloves of garlic a day.

A douche for vaginal thrush may help relieve symptoms. Place 30ml of white vinegar, the contents of two acidophilus capsules, 3 drops of tea-tree oil and 1 cup of warm water in a 'squeezy' plastic sauce bottle. Use each night or morning for 3 days before showering but don't use during your period.

Menu choices

These recipes offer a combination of ideal foods for candida.

Breakfast
Protein shake
Poached eggs with spinach & yoghurt (yeast-free bread)
Sardines & tomato on toast

Lunch
Tuna salad
Mediterranean salad
Lentil salad
Spanish omelette with feta & dill
Beef salad
Pea soup
Minestrone with pesto
Carrot & ginger soup with coriander

Dinner
Flathead fillets with potato & herb salad
Moroccan lamb with couscous
Marlin with green beans, pesto & roast tomatoes
Roast lamb with root vegetables
Spaghetti with chicken, cherry tomatoes, basil & pine nuts
Lamb cutlets with mashed potato, garlic green beans & roast tomatoes
Almost shepherd's pie
Veal shanks
Chilli con carne with avocado & yoghurt topping
Garlic prawns
Mediterranean fish soup
Lentil stew

Snack
Eggplant & tahini dip
Beetroot & yoghurt dip
Chickpea & tahini dip
Rice paper rolls
Spicy avocado mash on garlic toast (yeast-free bread)

Treat
Pumpkin & pepita muffins

Drink
Iced spiced green tea
Peppermint tea with ginger

Juice companions

Try carrot, celery, parsley, beetroot or spinach added to your favourite base juice. No sweet fruit juice.

Circulation, poor

What to eat

Buckwheat, rye, ginger, chillies, garlic, pith of citrus fruits, basil, cinnamon, curries, cherries, blueberries and blackberries.

What to avoid

Alcohol, sugar and white flour products.

Home help

If you feel the cold, eat more grounding and warming foods, such as curries, baked dinners and stewed fruits (especially during winter), rather than lighter, cooler foods, such as salads, stir-fries and raw fruit. Regular exercise is also important.

Menu choices

These recipes offer a combination of ideal foods for poor circulation, cold hands and feet, chill-blains, varicose veins and Raynaud's syndrome.

Breakfast
Porridge
Baked brown rice pudding with apricots

Lunch
Spanish omelette
Beef salad
Pea soup
Steak sandwich with horseradish cream & snow pea sprouts
Red lentil soup
Carrot & ginger soup with coriander

Dinner
Honey & soy chicken with rice
Moroccan lamb with couscous
Roast lamb with root vegetables
Lamb cutlets with mashed potato, garlic green beans & roas tomatoes
Roast beef with mustard, chives & garlic
Almost shepherd's pie

Chilli con carne with avocado & yoghurt topping
Braised beef with red wine & herbs
Chickpea curry
Garlic prawns
Lentil stew

Treat
Apple & blackberry crumble
Chocolate & raspberry muffins
Mixed berries in blackcurrant jelly

Drink
Hot cocoa
Iced lemongrass tea
Iced spiced green tea
Pear & ginger juice
Vegetable cocktail
Spiced tomato juice

Juice companions

Try ginger, beetroot, spinach, berries or grapefruit added to your favourite base juice.

Colds

What to eat

Chicken soup, chilli, ginger, garlic, carrots, cabbage, broccoli, parsley, basil, onions, miso, lemons, oranges, thyme, cloves, cinnamon, raw honey and nasturtiums, plus 3 litres of fluid daily (water, tea or soup).

What to avoid

While symptoms persist, milk products, alcohol and sugar.

Home help

In a teapot or plunger, combine the juice of 1 lemon, the rind of ½ of the lemon, ½ a stick of cinnamon, ½ bunch of thyme, 3cm of fresh ginger root grated and raw honey to taste. Add boiling water and stand for 5 minutes. Drink 3–6 cups of this tea every day of the cold.

Menu choices

These recipes offer a combination of ideal foods for colds.

Breakfast
Mango, banana & tofu smoothie

Lunch
Mediterranean salad
Spanish omelette
Red lentil soup
Carrot & ginger soup with coriander

Dinner
Honey & soy chicken with rice
Moroccan lamb with couscous
Almost shepherd's pie
Chilli con carne with avocado & yoghurt topping
Veal shanks
Chickpea curry
Mediterranean fish soup
Lentil stew

Snack
Spicy avocado mash on garlic toast

Treat
Mixed berries in blackcurrant jelly (no cream)
Apricot & tofu pudding

Drink
Lemonade with mint leaves
Pear & ginger juice
Carrot, apple & orange juice

Juice companions

Try orange, lemon, pineapple, carrot or ginger added to your favourite base juice.

Cold sores

What to eat

Fish, shellfish, bean sprouts, fruit, vegetables, oats, legumes.

What to avoid

Peanuts, almonds, hazelnuts, pecans, sesame seeds, walnuts, bacon, chocolate, sugar, carob, coconut, soy.

Home help

Rinsing the site with diluted apple cider vinegar can reduce the pain of a herpes outbreak and help dry out the sores. Dabbing with aloe vera gel will help them to heal.

Menu choices

These recipes offer a combination of ideal foods for cold sores and other herpes, including shingles, genital herpes and chicken pox.

Breakfast
Porridge
Protein shake
Mango, banana & tofu smoothie
Sardines & tomato on toast

Lunch
Tuna salad
Mediterranean salad
Lentil salad
Minestrone with pesto

Dinner
Flathead fillets with potato
  & herb salad
Marlin with green beans, pesto
  & roast tomatoes
Chilli con carne with avocado
  & yoghurt topping
Great northern beans with rice
Garlic prawns
Mediterranean fish soup

Snack
Eggplant & tahini dip
Beetroot & yoghurt dip
Chickpea & tahini dip

Treat
Pumpkin pudding with nutmeg
  & walnuts

Drink
Carrot, apple & orange juice

Juice companions

Try lemon, orange, carrot, celery, parsley or spinach added to your favourite base juice.

Constipation

What to eat

Choose wholegrain products where possible (eg, brown rice and wholemeal bread), beetroot, legumes, pears, oranges, prunes, green leafy vegetables, olive oil, nuts (daily), figs, buckwheat, coriander, green beans, cabbage and vegetable juice with beetroot, plus drink 2 litres water daily.

What to avoid

Red meat, sugar, chocolate, white flour products and yellow cheese.

Home help

Drink the juice of ½ a lemon in hot water first thing each morning to help get things moving. A strong cup of coffee will also help, as caffeine is a smooth muscle relaxant.

Menu choices

These recipes offer a combination of ideal foods for constipation.

Breakfast
Porridge
Bircher muesli
Toasted muesli with yoghurt
Baked brown rice pudding with apricots

Lunch
Mediterranean salad
Lentil salad
Pea soup
Minestrone with pesto
Zucchini slice
Brown rice & tuna salad
Red lentil soup

Dinner
Almost shepherd's pie
Chilli con carne with avocado & yoghurt topping
Chickpea curry
Great northern beans with rice
Lentil stew

Snack
Eggplant & tahini dip
Beetroot & yoghurt dip
Chickpea & tahini dip
Rice paper rolls
Spicy avocado mash on garlic toast

Treat
Apple & blackberry crumble
Poached pears with chocolate sauce
Stewed apricots with honey yoghurt & almonds
Pumpkin & pepita muffins
Oat & sunflower-seed cookies
Apple & blueberry muffins

Drink
Pear & ginger juice
Vegetable cocktail

Juice companions

Try spinach, pear or beetroot added to your favourite base juice.
Sip lemon juice, mixed with hot water, in the mornings.

Cystitis

What to eat

Blueberries, cranberries, unsweetened cranberry juice, asparagus, garlic, onions, leeks, parsley, celery, yoghurt, miso soup, zucchini, green beans and avocado, and juices, including celery and parsley. Plus 3 litres water daily.

What to avoid

In general, reduce yeast in your diet and avoid sugar. During a bout of cystitis, avoid red meat, sugar, yeast, caffeine, alcohol, chocolate and white flour products.

Home help

Barley water is a wonderful soother when you have cystitis. Simmer 50g of pearl barley in 1 litre of water until reduced by half. Drink this with a little raw honey, if desired.

Menu choices

These recipes offer a combination of ideal foods for cystitis.

Breakfast

Protein shake
Scrambled eggs with basil
   (yeast-free bread)
Poached eggs with spinach & yoghurt
Sardines & tomato on toast
   (yeast-free bread)

Lunch

Tuna salad
Mediterranean salad
Lentil salad
Omelette with feta & dill
Spanish omelette
Beef salad
Pea soup
Minestrone with pesto
Brown rice & tuna salad

Dinner

Zucchini slice
Flathead fillets with potato
   & herb salad
Moroccan lamb with couscous
Marlin with green beans, pesto
   & roast tomatoes
Roast lamb with root vegetables
Lamb cutlets with mashed potato, garlic
   green beans & raos tomatoes
Almost shepherd's pie

Chilli con carne with avocado
   & yoghurt topping
Chickpea curry
Garlic prawns
Lentil stew

Snack

Pumpkin & pepita muffins
Eggplant & tahini dip
Beetroot & yoghurt dip
Chickpea & tahini dip
Rice paper rolls
Spicy avocado mash on garlic toast
   (yeast-free bread)

Treat

Mixed berries in blackcurrant jelly
Apricot & tofu pudding

Drink

Iced lemongrass tea
Ayran
Vegetable cocktail

Juice companions

Try all berries (especially cranberries), carrot, celery or cucumber added to your favourite base juice.

Diabetes NIDDM (mature onset diabetes)

What to eat

Legumes, globe artichokes, Jerusalem artichokes, onions, fenugreek, quinces, berries, meat, fish, chicken, nuts, seeds and vegetables. See Antioxidants p183.

What to avoid

Sugar, soft drinks, white flour products, dried fruits, caffeine and juices.

Home help

Eat a small meal every 2–3 hours. Each meal should contain protein the size of your palm for a main meal, and half a palm for snacks.

Fenugreek helps stabilise blood sugar levels. Drink a cup of fenugreek tea once or twice daily—place 1 teaspoon of fenugreek seeds in a cup and add boiling water. A teaspoon of raw honey may be added for taste—honey doesn't affect blood sugar levels as severely as sugar (sucrose).

Menu choices

These recipes offer a combination of ideal foods for mature onset diabetes.

Breakfast
Porridge
Protein shake
Scrambled eggs with basil
Eggs with tomato, feta & herbs
Poached eggs with spinach & yoghurt
Sardines & tomato on toast

Lunch
Tuna salad
Mediterranean salad
Lentil salad
Omelette with fetta & dill
Spanish omelette
Beef salad
Pea soup
Minestrone with pesto
Zucchini slice
Red lentil soup

Dinner
Moroccan lamb with couscous
Marlin with green beans, pesto & roast tomatoes
Lamb cutlets with mashed potato, garlic green beans & roast tomatoes
Roast beef with mustard, chives & garlic
Almost shepherd's pie
Chilli con carne with avocado & yoghurt topping
Braised beef with mushrooms, red wine & herbs
Veal shanks
Garlic prawns
Great northern beans with rice
Lentil stew

Snack
Pumpkin & pepita muffins
Eggplant & tahini dip
Beetroot & yoghurt dip
Chickpea & tahini dip
Rice paper rolls
Spicy avocado mash on garlic toast

Treat
Ricotta cheesecake
Apricot & tofu pudding
Oat & sunflower-seed cookies

Juice companions

Try carrot or celery added to your favourite base juice. Dilute any fruit juice.

Diarrhoea

What to eat

Water, white rice, steamed chicken breast, white fish, tofu, vegetable broth, ginger, cooked pumpkin and carrot, mint, weak black or green tea, blueberries, cinnamon and mashed banana.

What to avoid

Fatty foods, milk products (except a little yoghurt), fruit juice, avoid, green vegetables and chilli.

Home help

Grate 1 peeled apple and leave it to turn brown before eating.

Menu choices

These recipes offer a combination of ideal foods for diarrhoea. Dehydration is a risk with diarrhoea, drink plenty of fluids. Eat only small portions. If the food causes more diarrhoea, desist. White rice and/or plain white toast are the first foods to try. If diarrhoea, persists seek medical assistance.

Lunch
Pea soup

Dinner
Flathead fillets with potato
    & herb salad
Honey & soy chicken with rice
    (no chilli)
Marlin with green beans
    & roast tomatoes (no pesto)

Snack
Pumpkin & pepita muffins

Treat
Mixed berries in blackcurrant jelly
    (no cream)
Apple & walnut pie
Pumpkin pudding with nutmeg
    & walnuts
Poached pears with chocolate sauce
    (no sauce)
Apricot & tofu pudding
Stewed apricots with honey yoghurt
    & almonds

Drink
Iced lemongrass tea
Iced spiced green tea
Pear and ginger juice
    (dilute ½ with water)
Peppermint tea with ginger

Juice companions

Try diluted apple or pear juice or ginger added to your favourite base juice.

Eczema

What to eat

Fish, carrots, avocados, nuts, seeds, tahini, walnuts, oats, olive oil and carrot juice, plus 10ml flaxseed oil daily, added to salad dressing or drizzled over vegetables.

What to avoid

Sugar and alcohol, and reduce red meat. Trigger foods may include wheat, milk, eggs, peanuts and food additives.

Home help

Avoid soap, use an oat 'sock' instead. Cut some old pantihose into 20cm lengths. Tie a knot at one end and fill with a couple of handfuls of rolled oats, tie a knot at the other end and use in bath or shower instead of soap. Hint, they only last one bath or shower, so make a few to last.

Menu choices

These recipes offer a combination of ideal foods for eczema, dermatitis and dry skin.

Breakfast
Porridge
Toasted muesli with yoghurt
Mango, banana & tofu smoothie
Sardines & tomato on toast

Lunch
Tuna salad

Dinner
Flathead fillets with potato & herb salad
Marlin with green beans, pesto & roast tomatoes
Garlic prawns
Mediterranean fish soup

Snack
Chickpea & tahini dip
Spicy avocado mash on garlic toast

Treat
Pumpkin pudding with nutmeg & walnuts
Apricot & tofu pudding
Stewed apricots with honey yoghurt & almonds
Oat & sunflower-seed cookies

Drink
Iced lemongrass tea
Vegetable cocktail

Juice companions

Try apricots, pear, apple, carrot, beetroot, celery or parsley added to your favourite base juice.

Eye health

What to eat

Turmeric, cocoa, all fruit and vegetables (especially carrots), chilli, ginger, parsley, berries (especially blueberries), and tomatoes.

What to avoid

Sugar, artificial sweeteners, margarine and processed oils (ie, not cold-pressed).

Home help

Placing a cold used tea bag over each eye for about 10 minutes reduces puffiness, redness and swelling.

Menu choices

These recipes offer a combination of ideal foods for eye health, including prevention of cataracts and macular degeneration.

Breakfast

Toasted muesli with yoghurt
Mango, banana & tofu smoothie (add berries)
Fruit salad with mint & yoghurt
Baked brown rice pudding with apricots
Poached eggs with spinach & yoghurt
Eggs with tomato, feta & herbs
Sardines & tomato on toast

Lunch

Tuna salad
Mediterranean salad
Lentil salad
Spanish omelette
Beef salad
Red lentil soup
Carrot & ginger soup with coriander

Dinner

Moroccan lamb with couscous
Marlin with green beans, pesto & roast tomatoes
Almost shepherd's pie
Chilli con carne with avocado & yoghurt topping
Chickpea curry
Mediterranean fish soup
Lentil stew

Snack

Beetroot & yoghurt dip

Treat

Chocolate polenta cake with choc chips
Mixed berries in blackcurrant jelly
Pumpkin pudding
Stewed apricots with honey yoghurt & almonds
Apricot & tofu pudding
Apple & blueberry muffins
Chocolate & raspberry muffins

Drink

Hot cocoa
Iced spiced green tea
Vegetable cocktail

Juice companions

Try apricots, berries (especially blueberries), rockmelon, beetroot or carrot added to your favourite base juice.

Gluten intolerance & coeliac disease

What to eat

All fruit, vegetables, meat, fish, eggs, legumes, nuts, seeds, yoghurt and grains—rice, corn, buckwheat, millet.

What to avoid

Gluten, wheat (bulgar, durum, bread flour, baker's flour, wholemeal flour and couscous), spelt, rye, oats, barley, triticale. Go easy on milk products except a little yoghurt.

Home help

Removing gluten from your diet also means the removal of fibre, which may result in constipation. Increase your intake of soluble fibre foods, including vegetables, legumes, nuts and seeds.

Menu choices

The majority of the recipes and menus suggested in this book, except those containing gluten, would be appropriate for anyone suffering from gluten intolerance and coeliac disease. For those recipes that suggest bread or pasta, use rice or a gluten-free substitute. Check that the sauces you use are gluten free.

Breakfast
Mango, banana & tofu smoothie
Fruit salad with mint & yoghurt
Scrambled eggs with basil

Lunch
Mediterranean salad
Omelette with fetta & dill
Pea soup
Minestrone with pesto

Dinner
Flathead fillets with potato & herb salad
Marlin with green beans, pesto & roast tomatoes
Almost shepherd's pie
Braised beef with red wine & herbs
Mediterranean fish soup

Snack
Beetroot & yoghurt dip
Rice paper rolls

Treat
Mixed berries in blackcurrant jelly
Poached pears with chocolate sauce
Ricotta cheesecake

Drink
Iced lemongrass tea
Iced spiced green tea
Ayran
Peppermint tea with ginger
Carrot, apple & orange juice
Vegetable cocktail

Juice companions

All juices.

Gum disease

What to eat

Raw fruit (especially citrus) and vegetables (especially carrots), thyme, sage, garlic, cloves and berries.

What to avoid

Sugar and white flour products.

Home help

Chewing food vigorously, especially crunchy raw fruit, vegetables, nuts and seeds, increases blood flow to the gums and increases the flow of saliva, which is antibacterial.

Eating a piece of aged cheddar after lunch or dinner also helps inactivate the bacteria behind gum disease.

Menu choices

These recipes offer a combination of ideal foods for gum disease, gingivitis and peridontal disease.

Breakfast
Toasted muesli with yoghurt
Fruit salad with mint & yoghurt
Eggs with tomato, feta & herbs

Lunch
Tuna salad
Mediterranean salad
Lentil salad
Red lentil soup
Carrot & ginger soup with coriander

Dinner
Moroccan lamb with couscous
Roast lamb with root vegetables
Chilli con carne with avocado & yoghurt topping
Lentil stew

Snack
Beetroot & yoghurt dip
Rice paper rolls

Treat
Mixed berries in blackcurrant jelly
Pumpkin & pepita muffins
Oat & sunflower-seed cookies
Chocolate & raspberry muffins

Drink
Iced lemongrass tea
Lemonade with mint leaves
Iced spiced green tea
Carrot, apple & orange juice
Vegetable cocktail

Juice companions

Try berries, pineapple, lemon, grapefruit or orange added to your favourite base juice.

Hayfever & sinus

What to eat

Garlic, horseradish, fish, lemons, grapefruit, oranges, limes, berries, capsicum, broccoli, fenugreek, buckwheat, raw honey and onions.

What to avoid

Sugar, alcohol, milk, gluten, egg, nuts, wheat, soy, food additives, peanuts, yeast and chocolate.

Home help

The neti pot (shaped like a small teapot) is an ancient Indian implement used for clearing the sinuses. Warm, salty water is poured into one nostril and flows out the other. It sounds weird, but once you get the hang of it you'll be hooked.

Menu choices

These recipes offer a combination of ideal foods for hayfever and sinus.

Breakfast
Mango, banana & tofu smoothie
Fruit salad with mint & yoghurt

Lunch
Mediterranean salad
Lentil salad
Spanish omelette
Minestrone with pesto
Steak sandwich with horseradish cream & snowpea sprouts.
Red lentil soup
Carrot & ginger soup with coriander

Dinner
Honey & soy chicken with rice
Moroccan lamb with couscous
Roast lamb with root vegetables
Lamb cutlets with mashed potato, garlic green beans & roast tomatoes
Roast beef with mustard, chives & garlic
Almost shepherd's pie
Chilli con carne with avocado & yoghurt topping
Veal shanks
Chickpea curry
Garlic prawns
Mediterranean fish soup
Lentil stew

Snack
Eggplant & tahini dip
Spicy avocado mash on garlic toast
Chickpea & tahini dip

Treat
Mixed berries in blackcurrant jelly
Apple & walnut pie
Pumpkin pudding with nutmeg & walnuts
Apricot & tofu pudding
Stewed apricots with honey yoghurt & almonds
Pumpkin & pepita muffins

Drink
Iced lemongrass tea
Iced spiced green tea
Lemonade with mint leaves
Peppermint tea with ginger
Carrot, apple & orange juice

Juice companions

Try pineapple, ginger, carrot or lemon added to your favourite base juice.

Headache

What to eat

All fruits and vegetables, meats, legumes, nuts and seeds, fish, chicken and eggs.

What to avoid

Coffee (beware of the caffeine withdrawal headache if you suddenly go off coffee). Triggers may include red wine, aged cheese, deli meats and smoked food, oranges, chocolate, aspartame and food additives.

Home help

Headaches are often caused by several factors, including stress, hormones, sinus, back problems and low blood sugar.

For immediate relief, sit with your feet in a bowl of hot water with cold compresses on your forehead and neck. Make sure you drink at least 2 litres of water daily.

Menu choices

These recipes offer a combination of ideal foods for sufferers of headaches.

Breakfast
Toasted muesli with yoghurt
Protein shake
Mango, banana & tofu smoothie
Scrambled eggs with basil
Baked brown rice pudding with apricots
Poached eggs with spinach & yoghurt
Eggs with tomato, feta & herbs
Sardines & tomato on toast
English muffin with cottage cheese, tomato & avocado

Lunch
Tuna salad
Lentil salad
Beef salad
Pea soup
Minestrone with pesto

Dinner
Flathead fillet
Honey & soy chicken with rice
Moroccan lamb with couscous
Spaghetti and chicken, cherry tomatoes, basil & pine nuts
Lamb cutlets with mashed potato, garlic green beans & roast tomatoes
Penne and tuna
Braised beef with red wine & herbs
Veal shanks
Great northern beans with rice
Lentil stew

Snack
Eggplant & tahini dip
Beetroot & yoghurt dip
Chickpea & tahini dip
Oat & sunflower-seed cookies
Rice paper rolls
Spicy avocado mash on garlic toast

Treat
Apple & walnut pie
Apricot & tofu pudding
Pumpkin & pepita muffins

Drink
Lemonade with mint leaves
Iced spiced green tea
Peppermint tea with ginger
Vegetable cocktail

Juice companions

Try pineapple, pear, carrot, celery, beetroot or ginger added to your favourite base juice.

Heart disease—high blood pressure, high cholesterol & atherosclerosis

What to eat

Oats, brown rice, nuts, fish (four times a week), legumes, salads, garlic, green tea, low-fat meats (eg, chicken without skin), cocoa, celery, pear, buckwheat, rosemary and all fruits and vegetables.

What to avoid

Salt, butter and high-fat dairy foods, sugar, caffeine, excess alcohol, fatty and fried foods, margarine and preserved oils. Reduce red meat.

Home help

Studies have shown that eating 25g of tree nuts (eg, almonds and brazil nuts) a day can be as effective as taking statin (cholesterol lowering) drugs.

Menu choices

These recipes offer a combination of ideal foods for heart disease.

Breakfast

Porridge
Bircher muesli
Mango, banana & tofu smoothie
Fruit salad with mint & yoghurt
Poached eggs with spinach & yoghurt
Sardines & tomato on toast
Toasted English muffin cottage cheese & avocado

Lunch

Tuna salad
Lentil salad
Pea soup
Minestrone with pesto
Brown rice & tuna salad
Red lentil soup

Dinner

Flathead fillets with potato & herb salad
Honey & soy chicken with rice
Marlin with green beans, pesto & roast tomatoes
Spaghetti with chicken, cherry tomatoes, basil & pine nuts
Almost shepherd's pie
Chilli con carne with avocado & yoghurt topping
Penne with tuna, olives & capers
Veal shanks
Chickpea curry
Great northern beans with rice
Mediterranean fish soup
Lentil stew

Snack

Pumpkin & pepita muffins
Eggplant & tahini dip
Beetroot & yoghurt dip
Chickpea & tahini dip
Rice paper rolls

Treat

Mixed berries in blackcurrant jelly (no cream)
Apple & walnut pie
Pumpkin pudding
Ricotta cheesecake
Apricot & tofu pudding
Stewed apricots with honey yoghurt & almonds
Oat & sunflower-seed cookies
Chocolate & raspberry muffins

Drink

Hot cocoa
Iced spiced green tea
Vegetable cocktail

Juice companions

Try pear, apple, grapefruit, carrot, celery or cucumber added to your favourite base juice.

Immune system

What to eat

Whole grains, rolled oats, brown rice, wholemeal bread, avocados, nuts, berries, shiitake mushrooms, garlic, onions, fish, walnuts, mangoes, oranges, lemons, leeks, asparagus, carrots, brazil nuts, yoghurt, parsley, kale and celery.

What to avoid

White flour, sugar and alcohol.

Home help

Drink a vegetable cocktail daily and, add some wheat grass, if available. You need to be vigilant with your diet and drink 2 litres of water daily.

Menu choices

These recipes offer a combination of ideal foods for those with a tendency to infections.

Breakfast
Bircher muesli
Toasted muesli with yoghurt
Protein shake
Mango, banana & tofu smoothie
Fruit salad with mint & yoghurt
Poached eggs with spinach & yoghurt

Lunch
Tuna salad
Mediterranean salad
Lentil salad
Beef salad
Minestrone with pesto
Red lentil soup
Carrot & ginger soup with coriander

Dinner
Almost shepherd's pie
Chickpea curry
Great northern beans with rice
Lentil stew

Snack
Pumpkin & pepita muffins
Beetroot & yoghurt dip
Chickpea & tahini dip
Oat & sunflower-seed cookies
Rice paper rolls
Spicy avocado mash on garlic toast

Treat
Mixed berries in blackcurrant jelly
Pumpkin pudding

Drink
Lemonade with mint leaves
Iced spiced green tea
Carrot, apple & orange juice
Vegetable cocktail

Juice companions

Try beetroot, parsley, carrot, lemon, ginger, orange or berries added to your favourite base juice.

Inflammatory bowel disease

What to eat

Soups, ginger, mint, garlic, okra, oysters, yoghurt, apples, papaya, pineapple, miso, cabbage and oats.

What to avoid

Sugar, carrageenan (a thickening agent used in some dairy products) and spicy foods, (eg, pepper and chilli). While condition is inflamed, avoid raw vegetables, whole nuts and seeds, red meat and wheat bran. Trigger foods may include gluten, dairy, chocolate, corn, eggs and bananas.

Home help

To help reduce inflammation of the intestine, drink raw carrot and cabbage juice daily: 2/3 carrot, 1/3 cabbage. Dilute with water if necessary.

A high-fibre diet is terrific for the bowel, but when the bowel is very inflamed, stick to low-fibre or puréed food.

Menu choices

These recipes offer a combination of ideal foods for inflammatory bowel disease (colitis, crohns).

Breakfast
Porridge
Protein shake
Mango, banana & *tofu smoothie*
Fruit salad with mint & yoghurt

Lunch
Tuna salad
Mediterranean salad
Lentil salad
Omelette with feta & dill
Pea soup
Minestrone with pesto
Carrot & ginger soup with coriander (no chilli)

Dinner
Flathead fillets with potato & herb salad
Honey & soy chicken with rice (no chilli)
Marlin with green beans, pesto & roast tomatoes
Mediterranean fish soup

Snack
Pumpkin & pepita muffins
Eggplant & tahini dip
Beetroot & yoghurt dip
Chickpea & tahini dip
Chocolate & raspberry muffins

Treat
Apple & blackberry crumble
Mixed berries in blackcurrant jelly
Pumpkin pudding
Apricot & tofu pudding
Stewed apricots with honey yoghurt & almonds

Drink
Iced lemongrass tea
Iced spiced green tea
Pear & ginger juice
Aryan
Peppermint tea with ginger
Vegetable cocktail

Juice companions

Try pear, ginger or carrot added to your favourite base juice.

Insomnia

What to eat

Oats, legumes, eggs, tuna, chicken, pasta, apricots, lettuce, nuts, seeds, all fruit and vegetables, whole grains, basil, dill, soups and bananas.

What to avoid

Caffeine and a large meal within three hours of bedtime.

Home help

Sadly, supper is rarely taken nowadays. Eating a small meal (eg, soup or hot milk and honey before bed helps stabilise blood sugars throughout the night.

Before bed, drink Ayran (see p180,) or a cup of hot milk and honey with a dash of ground nutmeg. Milk contains the amino acid tryptophan, which converts to serotonin, the calming neurotransmitter; nutmeg has sedative properties.

Menu choices

These recipes offer a combination of ideal foods for insomnia.

Breakfast
Porridge
Baked brown rice pudding with apricots
Poached eggs with spinach & yoghurt
Eggs with tomato, feta & herbs
Toasted English muffin with cottage cheese, tomato & avocado

Lunch
Tuna salad
Beef salad
Pea soup
Minestrone with pesto

Dinner
Flathead fillets with potato & herb salad
Honey & soy chicken with rice
Marlin with green beans, pesto & roast tomatoes
Almost shepherd's pie
Penne with tuna, olives & capers
Mediterranean fish soup
Lentil stew

Snack
Pumpkin & pepita muffins
Eggplant & tahini dip
Beetroot & yoghurt dip
Chickpea & tahini dip

Treat
Apple and blackberry crumble
Mixed berries in blackcurrant jelly
Apple & walnut pie
Pumpkin pudding with nutmeg & walnuts
Poached pears with chocolate sauce
Ricotta cheesecake
Apricot & tofu pudding
Stewed apricots with honey yoghurt & almonds
Oat & sunflower-seed cookies
Chocolate & raspberry muffins

Drink
Ayran

Juice companions

Try pear, apple, berries or carrot added to your favourite base juice.

Irritable bowel syndrome

What to eat

Ginger, mint, yoghurt, oats, brown rice, fish, berries, apricots, mangoes, miso, cabbage and bananas.

What to avoid

Fried food and chewing gum. Trigger foods may include wheat, cocoa and sorbitol (an artificial sweetener).

Home help

Don't overload your digestive system with big meals. Eat your meals at the same time every day and make sure you chew each mouthful at least 6 or 7 times before swallowing.

Menu choices

These recipes offer a combination of ideal foods for irritable bowel syndrome.

Breakfast

Porridge
Bircher muesli
Protein shake
Mango, banana & tofu smoothie
Fruit salad with mint & yoghurt
Scrambled eggs with basil
Baked brown rice pudding with apricots

Lunch

Tuna salad
Lentil salad
Omelette with feta & dill
Pea soup
Minestrone with pesto
Zucchini slice
Carrot & ginger soup with coriander

Dinner

Flathead fillets with potato & herb salad
Honey & soy chicken with rice (no chilli)
Marlin with green beans, pesto & roast tomatoes
Mediterranean fish soup

Snack

Pumpkin & pepita muffins
Eggplant & tahini dip
Beetroot & yoghurt dip
Chickpea & tahini dip

Treat

Apple & blackberry crumble
Mixed berries in blackcurrant jelly
Pumpkin pudding
Apricot & tofu pudding
Stewed apricots with honey yoghurt & almonds
Chocolate & raspberry muffins

Drink

Iced lemongrass tea
Iced spiced green tea
Pear & ginger juice
Peppermint tea with ginger

Juice companions

Try pear, pineapple, ginger or mint added to your favourite base juice.

Lactose intolerance

What to eat

Small amounts of acidophilus yoghurt may be tolerated and some hard cheeses. All foods excluding milk products soy and rice milk are okay.

What to avoid

All animal milk products (cow, goat, sheep and buffalo) milk, cream, cheese, ice cream and yoghurt. Small amounts of yoghurt and butter may be tolerated.

Home help

If you need to avoid milk products then it's important to eat enough calcium-rich foods or take a calcium supplement.

Menu choices

The majority of the recipes and menus suggested in this book would be appropriate for the lactose intolerant. If you take care to avoid recipes that contain milk, cheese or large amounts of yoghurt. You can experiment and adapt most recipes by substituting these ingredients with soy or lactose-free milk products.

Breakfast
Bircher muesli
Toasted muesli with yoghurt
Protein shake (soy milk)
Eggs with tomato, feta & herbs
Sardines & tomato on toast
Toasted English muffin with cottage cheese, tomato & avocado

Lunch
Tuna salad
Lentil salad
Minestrone with pesto

Dinner
Marlin with green beans, pesto & roast tomatoes
Chickpea curry
Great northern beans with rice
Mediterranean fish soup
Lentil stew

Snack
Pumpkin & pepita muffins
Eggplant & tahini dip
Chickpea & tahini dip
Rice paper rolls

Treat
Apple & walnut pie
Pumpkin pudding
Apricot & tofu pudding
Oat & sunflower-seed cookies

Drink
Peppermint tea with ginger

Juice companions

All juices.

Menopause & osteoporosis

What to eat

Fish, miso, soy, seeds, legumes, sprouts, parsley, seaweed, nuts, green leafy vegetables, calcium-rich foods and broccoli.

What to avoid

Avoid tea and coffee for an hour after meals; spicy food, if suffering hot flushes; sugar and carbonated drinks, including soda water and excess alcohol.

Home help

For the hot flushes of menopause, which are often worse at night, before bed, sit with your feet in a bowl of cool water in which a few drops of peppermint oil has been added.

Menu choices

These recipes offer a combination of ideal foods for menopause and osteoporosis.

Breakfast
Bircher muesli
Toasted muesli with yoghurt
Protein shake (soy milk)
Mango, banana & tofu smoothie
Eggs with tomato, feta & herbs
Sardines & tomato on toast
Toasted English muffin with cottage cheese, tomato & avocado

Lunch
Tuna salad
Lentil salad
Minestrone with pesto

Dinner
Marlin with green beans, pesto & roast tomatoes
Chickpea curry
Great northern beans with rice
Mediterranean fish soup
Lentil stew

Snack
Pumpkin & pepita muffins
Eggplant & tahini dip
Chickpea & tahini dip
Rice paper rolls

Treat
Apple & walnut pie
Pumpkin pudding
Ricotta cheesecake
Apricot & tofu pudding
Oat & sunflower-seed cookies

Drink
Aryan
Peppermint tea with ginger

Juice companions

Try beetroot, cucumber, celery or rockmelon added to your favourite base juice.

Mouth ulcers

What to eat

Prevention: eggs, salmon, sardines, lentils, leafy green vegetables and seeds. During outbreak: eat cooling foods, such as pears, cucumbers, yoghurt, melons and mangoes.

What to avoid

Trigger foods may include wheat, gluten, tomatoes, dairy, nuts and fluoride toothpaste. Foods that irritate include tomatoes, vinegar, lemons and pineapple.

Home help

For relief, apply a paste of bicarbonate of soda and water directly onto the ulcer.

Menu choices

These recipes offer a combination of ideal foods for mouth ulcers.

Breakfast

Mango, banana & tofu smoothie
Fruit salad with mint & yoghurt
Scrambled eggs with basil

Lunch

Mediterranean salad
Omelette with fetta & dill
Pea soup
Minestrone with pesto

Dinner

Flathead fillets with potato
   & herb salad
Marlin with green beans, pesto
   & roast tomatoes
Almost shepherd's pie
Braised beef with red wine & herbs
Mediterranean fish soup

Snack

Beetroot & yoghurt dip
Rice paper rolls

Treat

Mixed berries in blackcurrant jelly
   (no cream)
Pumpkin pudding
Poached pears with chocolate sauce
Ricotta cheesecake
Apricot & tofu pudding

Drink

Iced lemongrass tea
Iced spiced green tea
Aryan
Peppermint tea with ginger
Carrot, apple & orange juice
Vegetable cocktail

Juice companions

Try cabbage, carrot, pear or rockmelon added to your favourite base juice. Avoid any juice that stings—eg, pineapple.

Nausea, morning sickness & travel sickness

What to eat

Ginger, diluted pear juice, steamed vegetables, miso, papaya, stewed fruit, cloves, mint, fruit, carrots, dry bread or crackers, rice and cinnamon.

What to avoid

Fatty foods and any foods that makes you feel nauseous.

Home help

Ginger is wonderful for nausea. Drink ginger tea or suck on crystallised ginger. For a short bout of vomiting or nausea, just keep your fluids up and eat nothing. However, if the nausea is chronic—morning sickness, motion sickness or chemotherapy—then it's important to eat small meals to maintain your blood sugar levels.

Menu choices

These recipes offer a combination of ideal foods for nausea and morning sickness and travel sickness.

Breakfast
Mango, banana & tofu smoothie
Fruit salad with mint & yoghurt

Lunch
Minestrone with pesto
Carrot & ginger soup with coriander (no coconut milk)

Dinner
Flathead fillets with potato & herb salad
Honey & soy chicken with rice
Marlin with green beans, pesto & roast tomatoes (no pesto)
Great northern beans with rice

Snack
Pumpkin & pepita muffins
Chocolate & raspberry muffins

Treat
Mixed berries in blackcurrant jelly (no cream)
Pumpkin pudding with nutmeg & walnuts
Apricot & tofu pudding

Drink
Iced lemongrass tea
Lemonade with mint leaves
Iced spiced green tea
Peppermint tea with ginger

Juice companions

Try pear, apple, ginger or carrot, added to your favourite base juice and diluted with water.

Overweight

What to eat

Fish, lean meat, chicken, eggs, legumes, all vegetables (except potatoes), fruit (except bananas), grapefruit, nuts and seeds.

What to avoid

White flour products, sugar, soft drinks and deep-fried food.

Home help

Keep your serving sizes small, especially the evening meal. Eat only one meal daily that contains starch (eg. bread, pasta, rice, potatoes, bananas and oats). Eat protein with every meal, including snacks, as this will reduce hunger pangs and increase metabolic rate.

Menu choices

These recipes offer a combination of ideal foods to help you manage your weight.

Breakfast
Bircher muesli
Protein shake (low-fat milk)
Mango, banana & tofu smoothie
Poached eggs with spinach & yoghurt
Sardines & tomato on toast
Toasted English muffin with cottage cheese, tomato & avocado

Lunch
Tuna salad
Mediterranean salad
Lentil salad
Omelette with feta & dill
Beef salad
Minestrone with pesto
Red lentil soup

Dinner
Honey & soy chicken with rice
Marlin with green beans, pesto & roast tomatoes
Almost shepherd's pie
Chilli con carne with avocado & yoghurt topping
Veal shanks
Chickpea curry
Great northern beans with rice
Mediterranean fish soup
Lentil stew

Snack
Beetroot & yoghurt dip
Rice paper rolls

Treat
Mixed berries in blackcurrant jelly
Apple & walnut pie
Apricot & tofu pudding
Stewed apricots with honey yoghurt & almonds
Chocolate & raspberry muffins

Drink
Iced spiced green tea

Juice companions

Try grapefruit, celery, beetroot, parsley, or cucumber added to your favourite base juice.

PMS & period problems

What to eat

Berries, seeds, nuts, legumes, soy, fish (four times a week), all fruit and vegetables, lean red meat, olive oil, whole grains and organic eggs.

What to avoid

Caffeine (especially 2 weeks before your period), sugar, salt, chocolate, white flour products, margarine and deep-fried food.

Home help

Try a ginger compress for period cramps. Place 1 cup of grated ginger in the middle of a kitchen wipe or tea towel. Fold to form a ginger parcel. Place in a shallow bowl and pour over 1 cup of boiling water. Leave until bearably hot. Gently squeeze and place on abdomen. Wrap your waist and ginger parcel with plastic wrap. Wrap again in a towel, lie down and keep warm for 20 minutes before unpeeling.

Menu choices

These recipes offer a combination of ideal foods for PMS and period problems.

Breakfast
Toasted muesli with yoghurt
Protein shake
Mango, banana & tofu smoothie
Eggs with tomato and fetta
Sardines & tomato on toast
Toasted English muffin with cottage cheese, tomato & avocado

Lunch
Tuna salad
Mediterranean salad
Minestrone with pesto

Dinner
Flathead fillets with potato & herb salad
Marlin with green beans, pesto & roast tomatoes
Chickpea curry
Great northern beans with rice
Mediterranean fish soup
Lentil stew

Snack
Eggplant & tahini dip
Beetroot & yoghurt dip

Treat
Apricot & tofu pudding
Pumpkin & pepita muffins
Oat & sunflower-seed cookies

Drink
Peppermint tea with ginger

Juice companions

Try celery, carrot, beetroot or parsley added to your favourite base juice.

Prostate

What to eat

Pepitas, fish, fresh berries (especially cranberries), cooked tomatoes and tomato products (eg, sauce and paste), oysters, redcurrants, blackcurrants, red grapefruit, cabbage, green beans, asparagus, barley, thyme and soy.

What to avoid

Margarine and reduce alcohol and caffeine.

Home help

Chew on a handful of pepitas every day.

Menu choices

These recipes offer a combination of ideal foods for an enlarged prostate and the prevention of problems.

Breakfast
Toasted muesli with yoghurt
Protein shake (soy milk)
Mango, banana & tofu smoothie
Sardines & tomato on toast

Lunch
Tuna salad
Lentil salad
Pea soup
Minestrone with pesto

Dinner
Marlin with green beans, pesto & roast tomatoes
Chilli con carne with avocado & yoghurt topping
Penne with tuna, olives & capers
Chickpea curry
Garlic prawns
Lentil stew
Great northern beans
Mediterranean fish soup

Snack
Apple & walnut pie
Pumpkin pudding
Chickpea & tahini dip
Oat & sunflower-seed cookies
Rice paper rolls

Treat
Mixed berries in blackcurrant jelly
Apricot & tofu pudding
Pumpkin & pepita muffins

Drink
Iced spiced green tea
Spicy tomato juice

Juice companions

Try celery, cucumber, parsley or carrot added to your favourite base juice.

Psoriasis

What to eat

Fish, nuts, seeds, beetroot, carrots, lemons, artichokes, brown rice, oats, avocados, leafy green vegetables, apricots, peaches, bitter lettuce (eg, radicchio and rocket), prunes.

What to avoid

Red meat, deli meats, pork, sugar, chocolate, alcohol (especially beer and wine), bread, yellow and blue cheese, mushrooms, yeast extracts, grapes, melons, dried fruit and margarine.

Home help

Get your skin wet with sea water as often as possible. If this isn't possible, have a sea-salt bath 2–3 times a week. Naturopaths believe that treating the liver helps with psoriasis. A reliable liver tonic is to drink lemon juice in hot water first thing each morning, adding honey to taste. Also aim to drink two litres of water daily.

Menu choices

These recipes offer a combination of ideal foods for psoriasis.

Breakfast
Porridge
Toasted muesli with yoghurt
Mango, banana & tofu smoothie
Sardines & tomato on toast

Lunch
Tuna salad
Brown rice & tuna salad
Minestrone with pesto

Dinner
Flathead fillets with potato & herb salad
Marlin with green beans, pesto & roast tomatoes
Garlic prawns
Mediterranean fish soup

Snack
Beetroot & yoghurt dip
Chickpea & tahini dip
Spicy avocado mash on garlic toast

Treat
Pumpkin pudding with nutmeg
Oat & sunflower-seed cookies

Drink
Vegetable cocktail

Juice companions

Try grapefruit, lemon, beetroot or carrot added to your favourite base juice.

Stress

What to eat

Oats, avocados, garlic, carrots, legumes, meat, chicken, fish, eggs, nuts, seeds, cheese, moderate alcohol, miso, apricots, bananas, plums, pears, onions, leeks, root vegetables, chamomile tea, dates, parsley, miso, basil and dill.

What to avoid

Caffeine, sugar and excess alcohol.

Home help

Learning to deal with life's stresses is paramount to good health. Do whatever it takes—exercise, counselling or meditation. Times of stress can cause people to under- or overeat, or eat the wrong foods. Remember, stress is bad enough for your health without poor eating habits; ensure you eat regular, nutritious meals. Soups and smoothies are excellent if stress affects your digestion.

Menu choices

These recipes offer a combination of ideal foods for stress-related conditions.

Breakfast
Porridge
Protein shake
Mango, banana & tofu smoothie
Scrambled eggs with basil
Baked brown rice pudding with apricots

Lunch
Poached eggs with spinach & yoghurt
Lentil salad
Omelette with feta & dill
Spanish omelette
Pea soup
Minestrone
Zucchini slice
Carrot & ginger soup with coriander

Dinner
Flathead fillets with potato & herb salad
Honey & soy chicken with rice
Marlin with green beans, pesto & roast tomatoes
Roast lamb with root vegetables
Almost shepherd's pie
Braised beef with red wine & herbs
Mediterranean fish soup
Lentil stew

Snack
Eggplant & tahini dip
Chickpea & tahini dip
Oat & sunflower-seed cookies
Rice paper rolls
Spicy avocado mash on garlic toast

Treat
Apple & walnut pie
Pumpkin pudding
Ricotta cheesecake
Apricot & tofu pudding
Stewed apricots with honey yoghurt & almonds
Pumpkin & pepita muffins

Drink
Peppermint tea with ginger
Iced lemongrass tea

Juice companions

Try carrot, pear, celery, pineapple or ginger added to your favourite base juice.

Tonsillitis & sore throat

What to eat

Onions, leeks, thyme, turmeric, sage, carrots, garlic, cinnamon, apricots, mangoes, blackberries, strawberries, lemons, legumes, miso, pineapple juice, honey and sage.

Foods to avoid

During an attack, avoid milk products and any foods that hurt to swallow.

Home remedies

In a teapot or plunger, add 1 teaspoon of the following: freshly chopped thyme and sage and freshly sliced ginger. Add boiling water, strain. Add honey and lemon to taste and sip 2 or 3 cups daily.

Menu choices

These recipes offer a combination of ideal foods for tonsillitis and sore throat.

Breakfast
Protein shake (soy/rice milk)
Mango, banana & tofu smoothie
Fruit salad with mint & yoghurt

Lunch
Spanish omelette
Pea soup
Minestrone with pesto
Red lentil soup
Carrot & ginger soup with coriander

Dinner
Marlin with green beans, pesto & roast tomatoes
Almost shepherd's pie
Chilli con carne with avocado & yoghurt topping
Chickpea curry
Mediterranean fish soup
Lentil stew

Snack
Eggplant & tahini dip
Beetroot & yoghurt dip
Chickpea & tahini dip
Chocolate & raspberry muffins

Treat
Mixed berries in blackcurrant jelly (no cream)
Apple & walnut pie
Pumpkin pudding with nutmeg
Poached pears with chocolate sauce
Ricotta cheesecake
Apricot & tofu pudding
Stewed apricots with honey yoghurt & almonds

Drink
Iced lemongrass tea
Lemonade with mint leaves
Iced spiced green tea
Pear & ginger juice
Carrot, apple & orange juice

Juice companions

Try pineapple, lemon or orange added to your favourite base juice.

The recipes

Gül McCarty

ALMOST SHEPHERD'S PIE	122
APPLE & BLACKBERRY CRUMBLE	140
APPLE & BLUEBERRY MUFFINS	166
APPLE & WALNUT PIE	145
APRICOT & TOFU PUDDING	153
AYRAN	180
BAKED BROWN RICE PUDDING WITH APRICOTS	61
BEEF SALAD	81
BEETROOT & YOGHURT DIP	161
BIRCHER MUESLI	53
BRAISED BEEF WITH MUSHROOMS, RED WINE & HERBS	125
BREAD PUDDING	155
BROWN RICE & TUNA SALAD	90
CARROT, APPLE & ORANGE JUICE	181
CARROT & GINGER SOUP WITH CORIANDER	93
CHICKPEA & TAHINI DIP	161
CHICKPEA CURRY	129
CHILLI CON CARNE WITH AVOCADO & YOGHURT TOPPING	123
CHOCOLATE & RASPBERRY MUFFINS	167
CHOCOLATE POLENTA CAKE WITH CHOC CHIPS	141
EGGPLANT & TAHINI DIP	159
EGGS WITH TOMATO, FETA & HERBS	65
FLATHEAD FILLETS WITH POTATO & HERB SALAD	108
FRUIT SALAD WITH MINT & YOGHURT	59
GARLIC PRAWNS	132
GREAT NORTHERN BEANS WITH RICE	133
HONEY & SOY CHICKEN WITH RICE	109
HOT COCOA	172
ICED LEMONGRASS TEA	173
ICED SPICED GREEN TEA	172
LAMB CUTLETS WITH MASHED POTATO, GARLIC GREEN BEANS & ROAST TOMATOES	120
LEMONADE WITH MINT LEAVES	173
LENTIL SALAD	76
LENTIL STEW	137
LUNCH BOXES	95
MANGO, BANANA & TOFU SMOOTHIE	58
MARLIN WITH GREEN BEANS, PESTO & ROAST TOMATOES	113
MEDITERRANEAN FISH SOUP	135
MEDITERRANEAN SALAD	73
MINESTRONE WITH PESTO	85
MIXED BERRIES IN BLACKCURRANT JELLY	144
MOROCCAN LAMB WITH COUSCOUS	112
OAT & SUNFLOWER-SEED COOKIES	162
OLIVE PASTE	161
OMELETTE WITH FETA & DILL	77
PEA SOUP	84
PEAR & GINGER JUICE	180
PENNE WITH TUNA, OLIVES & CAPERS	124
PEPPERMINT TEA WITH GINGER	181
POACHED EGGS WITH SPINACH & YOGHURT	64
POACHED PEARS WITH CHOCOLATE SAUCE	149
PORRIDGE	52
PROTEIN SHAKE	57
PUMPKIN & PEPITA MUFFINS	158
PUMPKIN PUDDING WITH NUTMEG & WALNUTS	148
RED LENTIL SOUP	92
RICE PAPER ROLLS	163
RICOTTA CHEESECAKE	152
ROAST BEEF WITH MUSTARD, CHIVES & GARLIC	121
ROAST LAMB WITH ROOT VEGETABLES	116
SARDINES & TOMATO ON TOAST	68
SCRAMBLED EGGS WITH BASIL	60
SPAGHETTI WITH CHICKEN, CHERRY TOMATOES, BASIL & PINE NUTS	117
SPANISH OMELETTE	80
SPICED TOMATO JUICE	184
SPICY AVOCADO MASH ON GARLIC TOAST	168
STEAK SANDWICH WITH HORSERADISH CREAM & SNOW PEA SPROUTS	88
STEWED APRICOTS WITH HONEY YOGHURT & ALMONDS	154
TOASTED ENGLISH MUFFINS WITH COTTAGE CHEESE, TOMATO & AVOCADO	69
TOASTED MUESLI WITH YOGHURT	56
TUNA SALAD	72
VEAL SHANKS	128
VEGETABLE COCKTAIL	184
ZUCCHINI SLICE	89

feelgood food

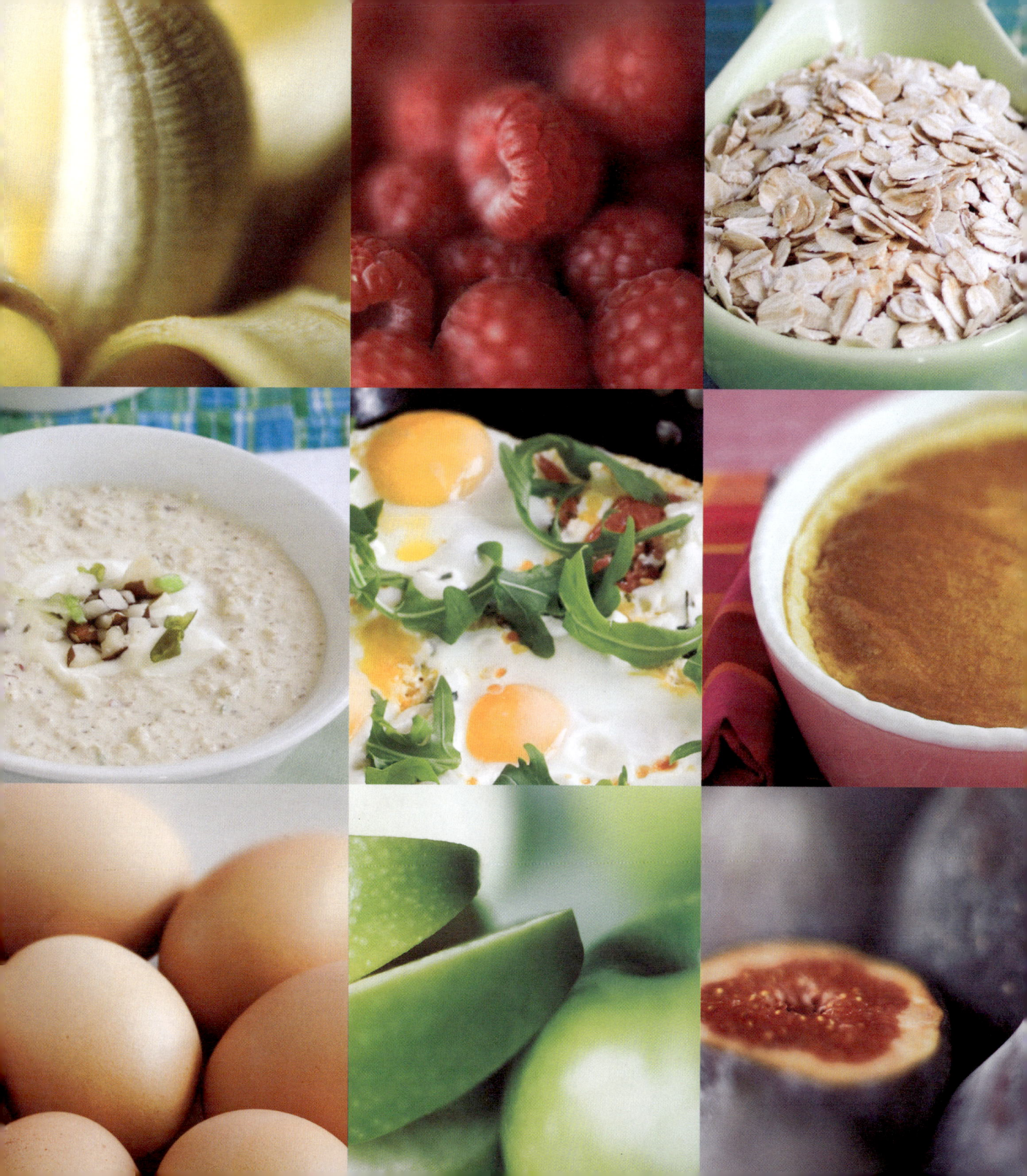

Breakfast

Given that the hours between dinner and breakfast are usually our longest without food, it's no wonder we often wake up ravenous. Whether it's a large bowl of cereal you crave or something involving eggs or sardines, on the pages that follow, you'll find delicious ideas for breaking your fast and fuelling your day. Remember, nothing prepares you better for the long hours ahead than a hearty morning meal; so don't eat on the run or, even worse, hang on until lunch time—as the old saying goes, 'breakfast like a king'.

PORRIDGE

This porridge is particularly good on a cold morning. It doesn't need sugar added to it, as grated pears and bananas provide enough sweetness. For those with gluten sensitivity, rolled oats can be replaced with rolled brown rice.

2 cups rolled oats
2 pears, grated
1 tablespoon shredded coconut
1 tablespoon LSA*
2 cups water
2 cups milk

TO SERVE
generous sprinkle of ground cinnamon
4 bananas, sliced
4 tablespoons chopped almonds or walnuts
4 teaspoons honey (optional)
2 cups milk, extra

Mix oats, pear, coconut, LSA, water and milk in a non-stick saucepan. Set aside for 15 minutes.

Cook on low heat for 15 minutes, stirring frequently.

Divide porridge between 4 bowls, sprinkle with cinnamon and add bananas, chopped nuts and honey, if using. Serve with extra milk.

SERVES 4

*LSA, a mixture of ground linseeds, sunflower seeds and almonds, is available from health food stores and supermarkets. It's best stored in an airtight container.

BIRCHER MUESLI

Bircher muesli will keep in the fridge, covered, for a couple of days.
If you don't want to use milk in the muesli, use fruit juice instead.

2 cups rolled oats
1 pear or apple, grated
$2/3$ cup natural yoghurt
$2/3$ cup milk
$2/3$ cup orange or apple juice
1 tablespoon LSA*
1 tablespoon honey (optional)

TO SERVE
2 tablespoons natural yoghurt
2 tablespoons chopped almonds

Combine oats, pear or apple, yoghurt, milk, juice, LSA and honey, if using, in a large bowl.

Cover and refrigerate overnight.

Serve with yoghurt and chopped almonds.

SERVES 4

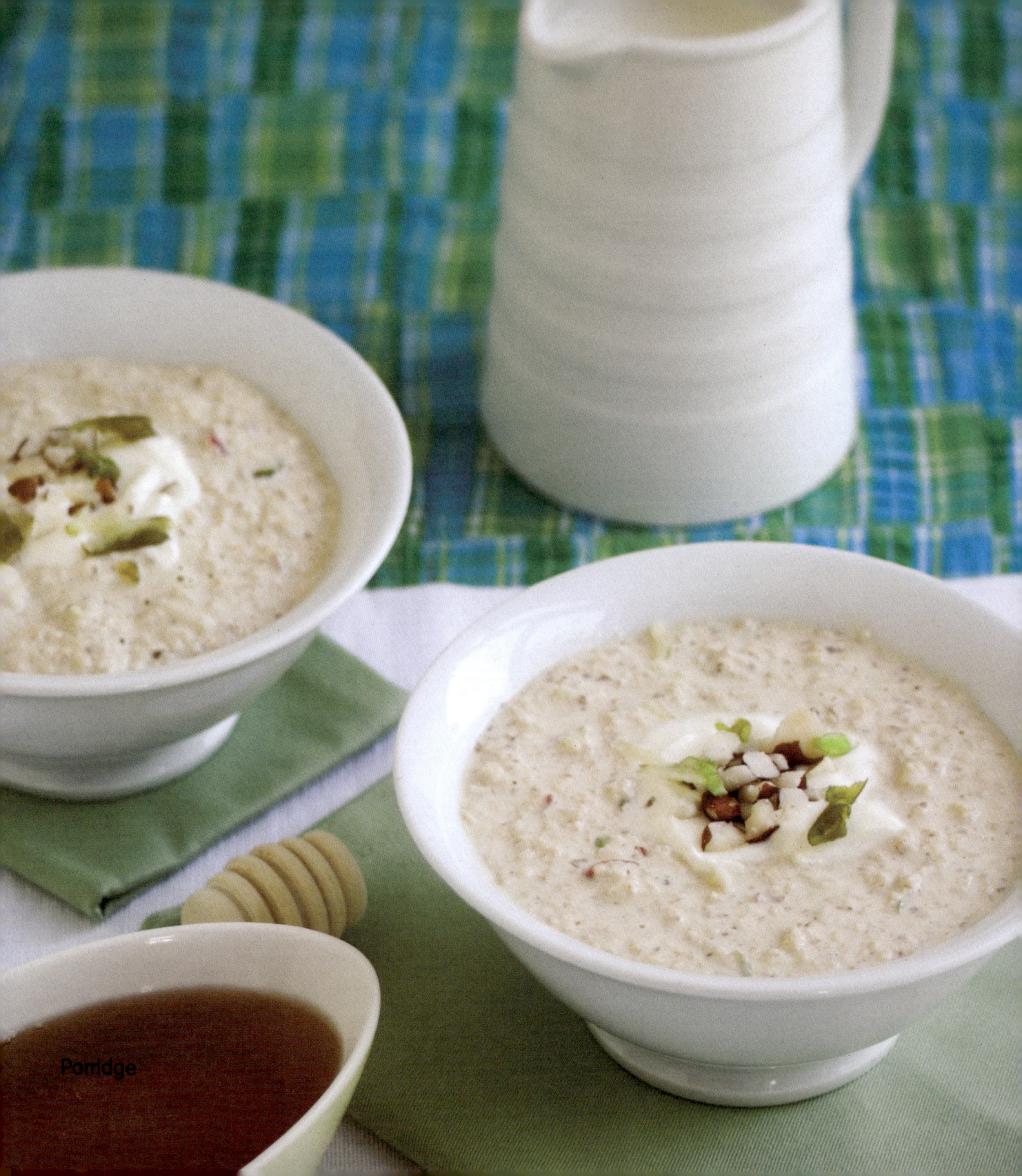

Porridge

Oats

Oats do wonders for the nervous system. After all, a nose-bag of oats is a traditional pep up for horses. Avenine, a substance in oats, is a nervous system tonic, making it as good for humans as it is for horses. Plus oats have the lowest glycaemic index (GI) of all grains. A low GI means blood sugar levels rise gradually and for a more sustained period, which is good news for diabetics and those with fluctuating blood sugar levels. It's also the reason why a bowl of porridge or muesli takes you further into the day than other breakfast cereals. Oats are highly recommended for those with high cholesterol because the fibre in them soaks up excess cholesterol and transports it out of the body. And they are astonishing rich in protein, calcium, potassium, magnesium and B-complex vitamins.

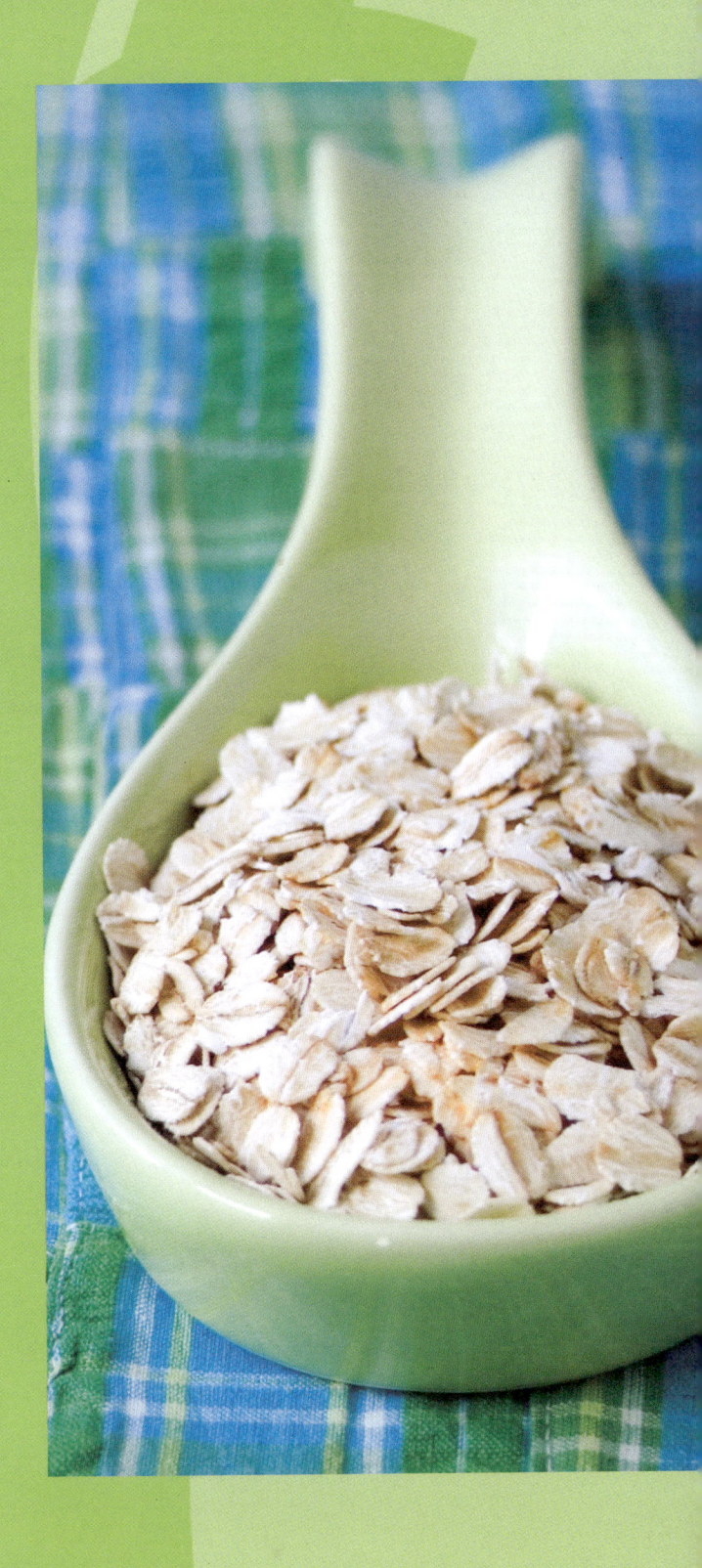

TOASTED MUESLI WITH YOGHURT

Why bother making your own toasted muesli when you can buy it? Because this one has no added oil or sugar, so it has to be better for you—and you can add to it or leave out anything you like. The quantities below will yield 12 cups of muesli—about 24 serves. It will keep in an airtight container for up to two months.

5 cups rolled oats
1 cup flaked almonds
1/3 cup sesame seeds
1 cup shredded coconut
1 cup dried apricots, diced
1 cup sultanas
1 cup sunflower seeds
1 cup pepitas

TO SERVE
2 cups natural yoghurt
2 cups berries of your choice
4 teaspoons honey (optional)

Preheat oven to 180°C/350°F.

Toast oats on an oven tray until golden brown (about 30 minutes). Toss oats after 15 minutes to ensure they toast evenly. Leave to cool on the tray.

Put almonds and sesame seeds in a non-stick frypan (don't add any oil). Stirring constantly, fry approximately 2 minutes, or until the almonds and sesame seeds turn. They cook very quickly, so don't leave them unattended. Transfer to the oven tray with the roasted oats.

Combine coconut, apricots, sultanas, sunflower seeds and pepitas with the oats, almonds and sesame seeds, and mix well.

Serve muesli with yoghurt, berries and honey, if using.

SERVES 24

PROTEIN SHAKE

This is my favourite breakfast during the week. It's fast, delicious and covers just about all major food groups. You won't be able to fit these quantities into your blender all at once, so mix it in two batches.

4 cups milk
8 tablespoons protein powder
2 tablespoons LSA*
4 bananas, chopped
2 cups berries (frozen or fresh) of your choice

Whizz all the ingredients in a blender until the mixture is smooth.

Pour into 4 large (600ml) glasses.

SERVES 4

MANGO, BANANA & TOFU SMOOTHIE

This is a variation on the Protein shake. Tofu provides the protein, and the fruit and fruit juice make a delicious refreshing drink that is totally satisfying, even without milk. Mix it in two batches.

4 mangoes (or 8 frozen mango cheeks)
4 bananas, chopped
4 cups orange juice
600g/1lb 5¼ oz silken tofu

Whizz all ingredients in a blender until smooth.

Pour into 4 large (600ml) glasses.

SERVES 4

FRUIT SALAD WITH MINT & YOGHURT

This is for those who don't really like breakfast—and also for lovers of fruit.

4 bananas, sliced
4 kiwi fruit, sliced
2 cups blueberries
2 oranges, diced
2 pears, diced
pulp of 4 passionfruit
½ cup chopped mint leaves

TO SERVE
2 cups natural yoghurt
1 tablespoon honey
2 tablespoons LSA

Combine fruit and mint leaves in a bowl.

Divide the fruit salad with mint and yoghurt between 4 bowls.

Mix yoghurt with honey and spoon over the fruit salad. Sprinkle each bowl with LSA.

SERVES 4

SCRAMBLED EGGS WITH BASIL

Eggs are a weekend affair in our house, but these scrambled eggs are quick enough to make during the week. If you are wondering about the cream, you can use milk instead but be warned: your eggs won't be as creamy and fluffy. If you do use cream, the eggs will taste so wonderful, you won't need any butter on your toast.

8 eggs
¾ cup fresh cream
1 cup basil leaves, chopped
2 tablespoons freshly grated Parmesan
sea salt and pepper

TO SERVE
8 slices sourdough bread, toasted

Combine eggs, cream, basil, Parmesan, and salt and pepper in a bowl and beat with a whisk.

Heat a large non-stick frypan over medium heat, pour in egg mixture. When mixture starts to set around the edges (about 2 minutes), give it a gentle stir in using a folding motion. Let it cook for another minute or two until the eggs are just set, then stir using a folding motion again.

Serve on hot toast.

SERVES 4

BAKED BROWN RICE PUDDING WITH APRICOTS

Serve this breakfast pudding at room temperature. It will keep in the fridge, covered, for two days. It can also double as a delicious dessert.

1½ cups brown rice
1½ cups water
12 dried apricots, diced
4 eggs
3 cups milk
1 tablespoon honey
2 teaspoons vanilla extract
grated zest of 1 orange

Cook rice in water and set aside. (This can be done the day before and stored in the fridge).

Preheat oven to 180°C/350°F.

Mix apricots with rice and transfer to an appropriate baking dish.

Beat eggs, milk, honey, vanilla and zest with an electric hand beater until honey dissolves.

Pour mixture over rice and apricots, and stir through.

Bake in oven until custard sets and the top turns golden brown (about 40 minutes).

Cool to room temperature.

SERVES 4

Baked brown rice pudding with apricots

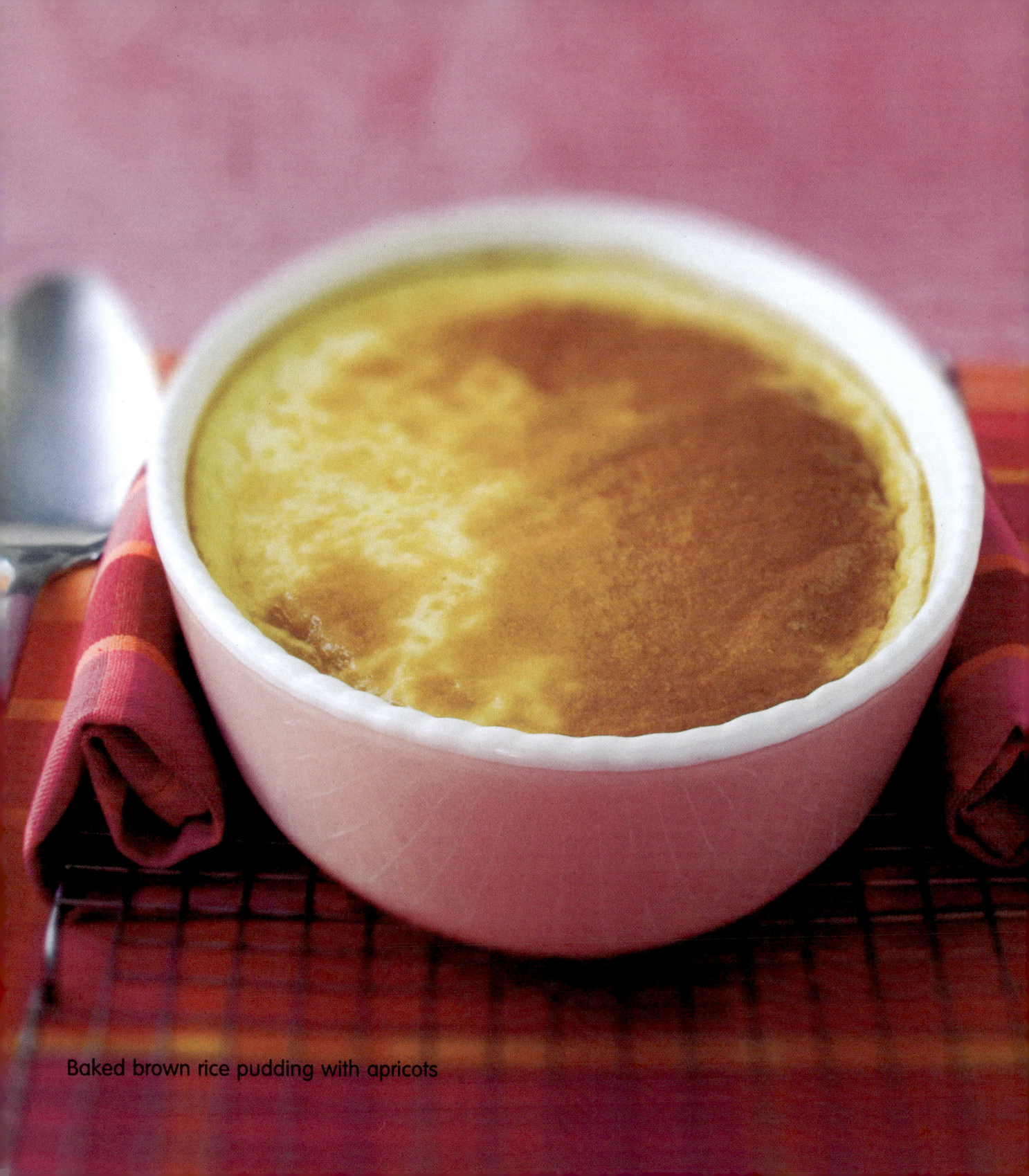

Eggs

Eggs are one of the best protein foods around. For millennia, they have been a prized food of humans and other animals, for good reason. In addition to protein (about 8g per egg), eggs are an excellent source of B12, iron, lecithin and vitamin A. They are also relatively low in fat. All in all, eggs are possibly the most nutritious of foods, gram for gram.

Unfortunately, in the past couple of decades, the egg has fallen from grace. This has been due mainly to the fear of cholesterol—high levels of cholesterol is, of course, one of the risk factors for heart disease. However, eating saturated fat from pastries, red meat, ice cream and cheese is much more likely to accelerate cholesterol levels than eating eggs. The lecithin in eggs helps in the metabolism of fats and cholesterol. Most people can eat an egg a day without any worry.

The best eggs to eat are those from hens that have been fed organic grains and vegetables.

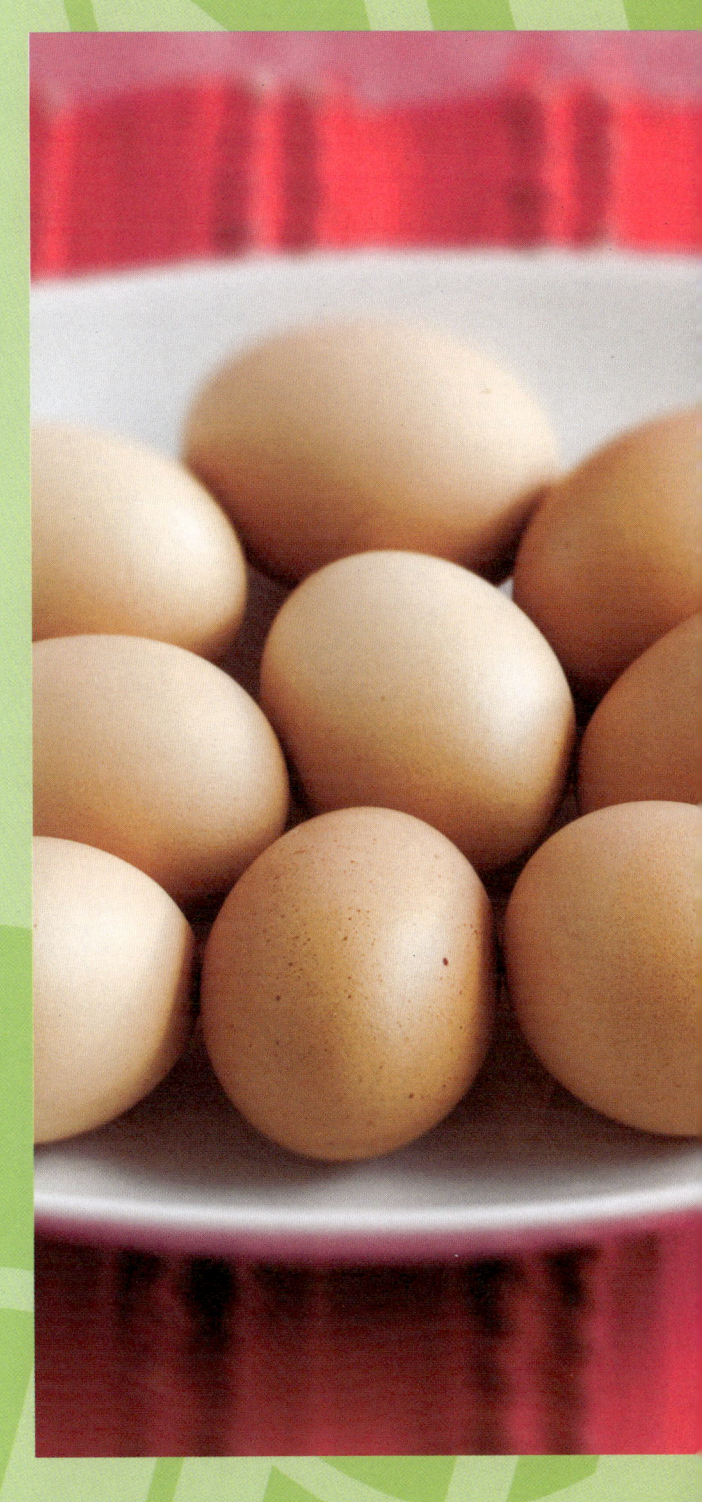

POACHED EGGS WITH SPINACH & YOGHURT

Garlic in the yoghurt might sound a bit strange to you, but where my family come from in Turkey, it's drizzled over most vegetables. Trust me, it's very good.

1 cup natural yoghurt
2 small garlic cloves, crushed (optional)
6 cups water
8 eggs, at room temperature
8 cups baby spinach leaves, washed
8 thick slices wholemeal bread
sea salt and pepper
chilli powder

Put yoghurt in a bowl, add garlic, if using, and whisk a little so to thin. Put aside.

Bring water to the boil in a deep frypan with a lid, then remove from heat. Reduce heat to low. Break eggs quickly into water, cover tightly with lid, and return to heat. Simmer very gently for 3 minutes, or until the whites are just cooked.

Put spinach in a saucepan, cover with a lid and cook on moderate heat until the leaves wilt. (You don't need to add any water to the saucepan). In the meantime, toast bread.

Place two slices of toast on 4 dinner plates. Place wilted spinach on a clean tea towel, squeeze out excess water, then spread spinach evenly on toast.

Remove eggs from pan with a slotted spoon and rest the spoon on kitchen paper for a few seconds to drain off excess water. Place eggs on spinach-topped toast. Season with salt and pepper. Drizzle a little of the reserved yoghurt mixture over the eggs and sprinkle with chilli powder.

SERVES 4

EGGS WITH TOMATO, FETA & HERBS

This is my version of an old family favourite. I remember every Sunday the family used to get together for brunch and we'd have eggs, wood-fired bread, lots of black tea and home-made black cherry jam.

8 Roma tomatoes, sliced
1 tablespoon olive oil
2 tablespoons chopped oregano
1 cup crumbled feta
8 eggs
8 drops Tabasco
sea salt and pepper

TO SERVE
4 cups baby rocket leaves
1 tablespoon olive oil
squeeze of lemon juice
8 slices of sourdough bread, toasted

Place tomato slices in a large non-stick frypan, add olive oil and cook on medium heat until tomatoes are soft (about 4 minutes).

Add oregano and feta and continue to cook until the feta starts to melt.

Remove pan from the heat and break in eggs. Dot each egg with a drop of Tabasco and season with salt and pepper.

Return pan to the heat, cook eggs until the whites are just solid (about three minutes). To achieve this without overcooking the yolks, cover the frypan with a lid when the egg whites start to turn opaque.

While the eggs are cooking, toss rocket leaves with olive oil and lemon juice and divide between 4 dinner plates.

Toast bread and place on rocket leaves.
Top with eggs and serve.

SERVES 4

Eggs with tomato, feta and herbs

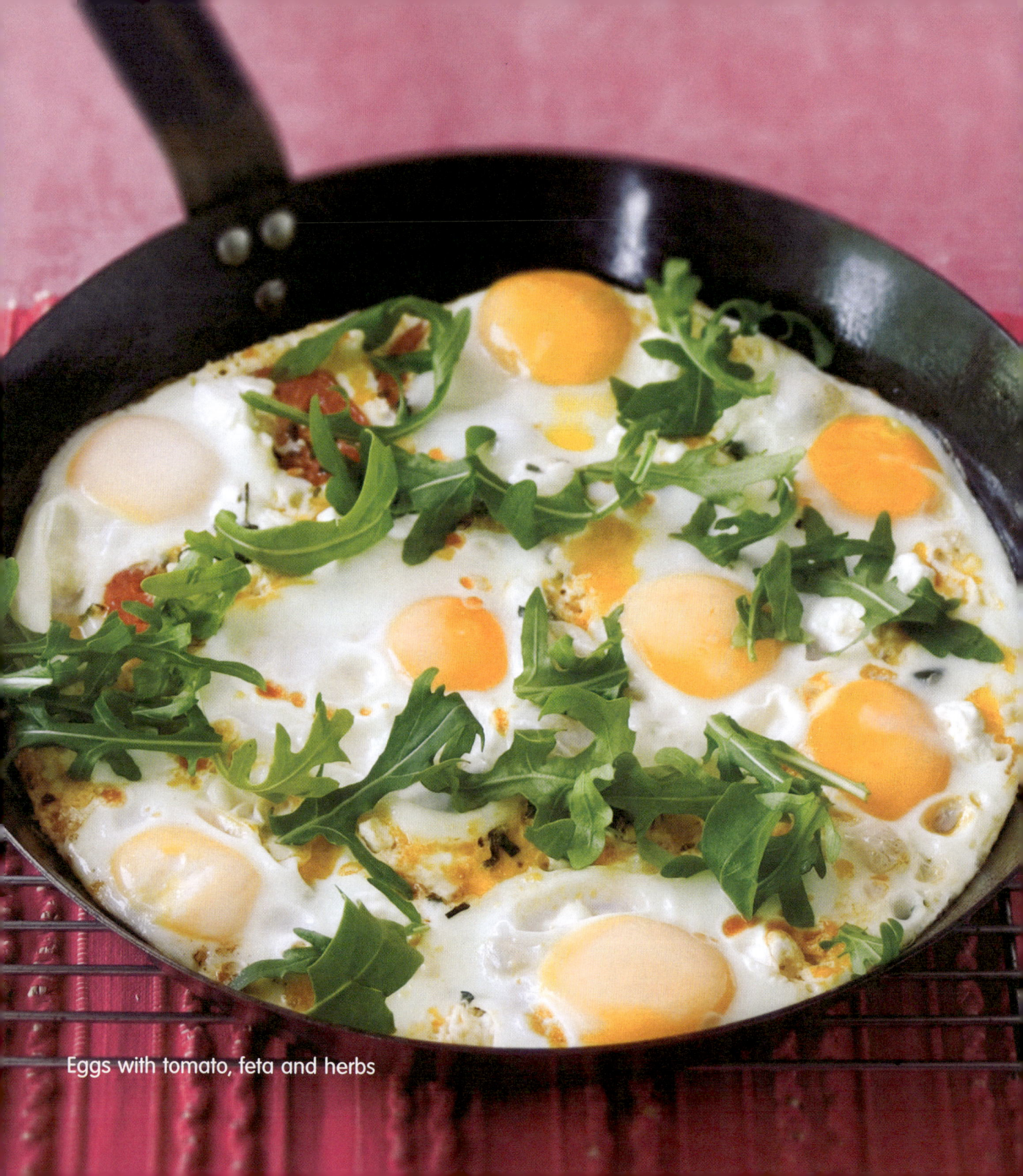

Calcium

Calcium makes up to 2 per cent of our body weight—that's about 1.2kg for a 60kg person. Ninety-nine per cent of calcium resides in our bones, where it adds strength to the protein matrix; the remaining 1 per cent helps regulate our heartbeat, contract muscles, clot blood and release nerve messengers. Because it's so vital for growing bodies, children require proportionately more calcium in their diet than adults. Loss of calcium from the bones is one of the causes of the bone-thinning disease osteoporosis. Unless we eat plenty of calcium-enhancing foods and exercise regularly, our bones start to thin from as early as our twenties.

Foods that are a good source of calcium include milk products (especially cheese), nuts, seeds, whole grains, figs, tofu, Asian greens, broccoli, carob, fish with edible bones (such as sardines, whitebait and canned salmon), tahini, seaweed, dried fruit, molasses, parsley, alfalfa and chickpeas. Foods that inhibit calcium absorption include salt, sugar, tea, coffee, excess red meat (that is, more than five times a week) and phosphates, which are mainly found in soft drinks. Aluminium-containing antacids also have a negative impact on calcium levels.

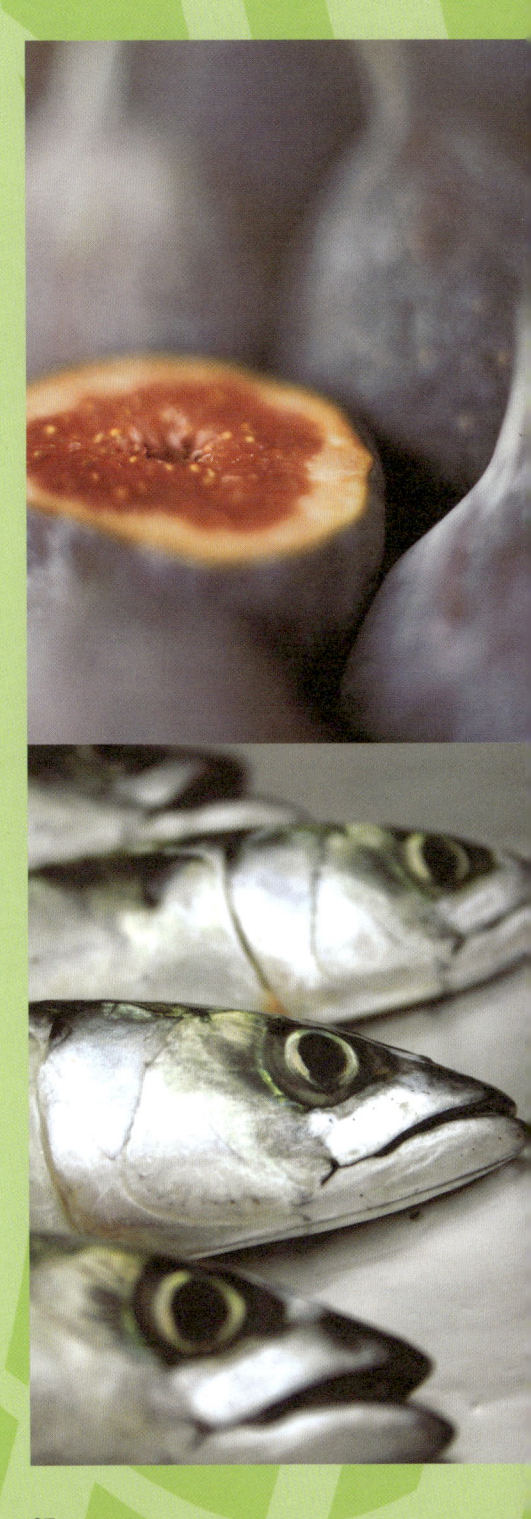

SARDINES & TOMATO ON TOAST

This could be rather challenging for young children to manage, so cut the toast into fingers and place a sardine on each one. Serve the tomato slices on the side. Always encourage children to eat fresh herbs. Start them with a sprig of dill on the tomato slices and try one yourself in front of them.

4 tomatoes, sliced
8 slices mixed-grain bread, toasted
sea salt and pepper
4 x 105g/3¾ oz cans sardines, drained well
2 tablespoons chopped dill
4 lemon wedges

Put slices of tomato on toast and sprinkle with sea salt.

Place sardines on tomato, sprinkle with pepper and dill and squeeze over lemon juice.

SERVES 4

TOASTED ENGLISH MUFFINS WITH COTTAGE CHEESE, TOMATO & AVOCADO

This breakfast qualifies as 'breakfast on the run', but it still provides all the nutrients your family needs for the morning. Young children might find it difficult to manage slices of tomato and avocado on the muffin, so mash the avocado for them and spread it under the cottage cheese, and serve the tomatoes on the side.

4 multigrain English muffins, cut in half	Toast muffins until golden.
4 tablespoons cottage cheese	
4 Roma tomatoes, sliced	Spread each muffin half with cottage cheese, then top with tomato and avocado slices.
2 avocados, sliced	
sea salt and pepper	
squeeze of lemon juice	Season with salt and pepper and add a squeeze of lemon juice.

SERVES 4

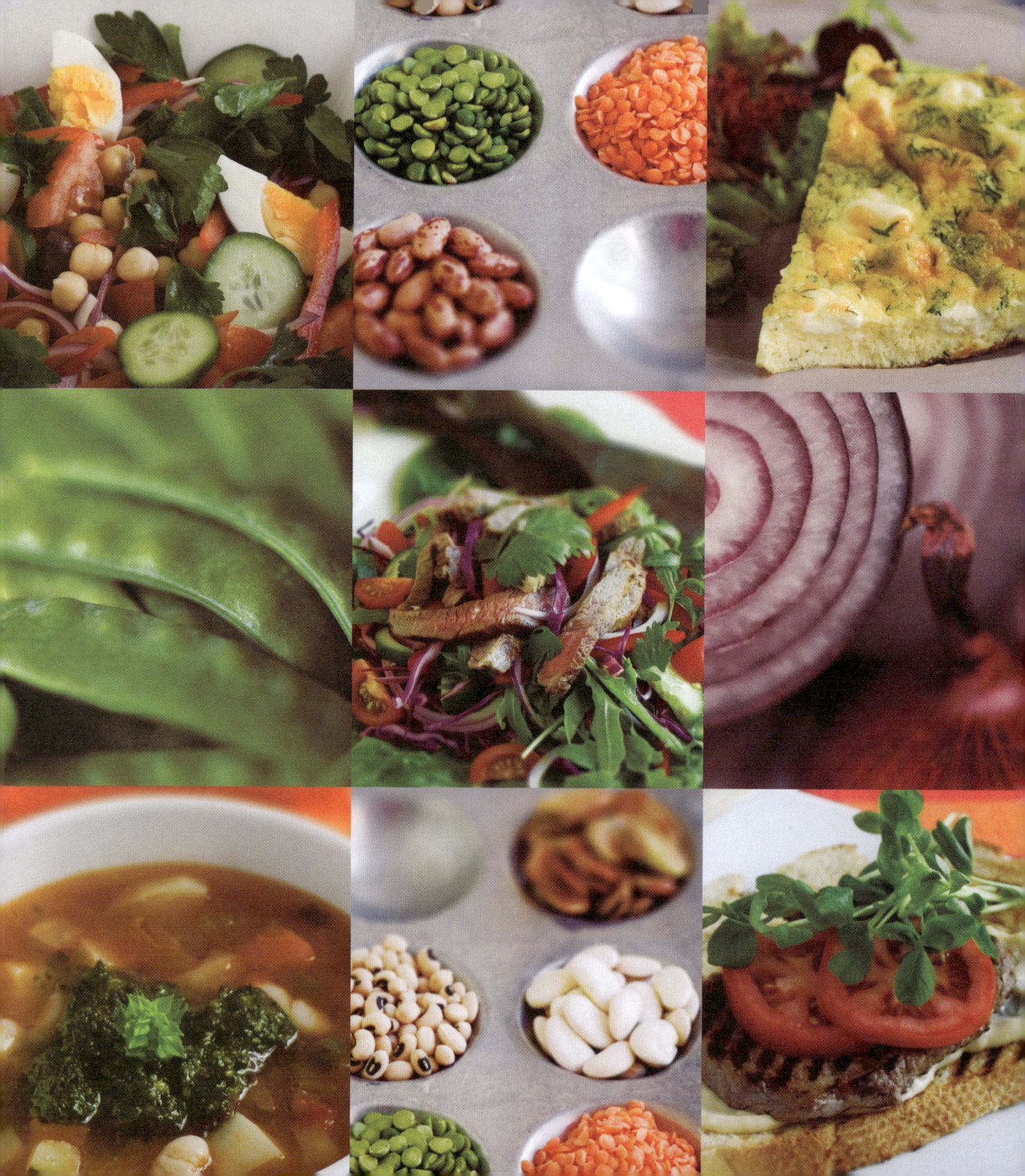

Lunch

While it's not possible for all members of the family to sit down and lunch together during the week, they can still eat the same lunch, whether from a lunchbox or on a plate. Of course, a few variations will be necessary to accommodate different requirements and portion sizes will vary, but one thing is for sure: everyone's lunch will be worth the wait. So toss the Vegemite and peanut butter sandwiches aside and treat your loved ones—big and small—to the tasty tucker on the following pages.

TUNA SALAD

This salad is easy to prepare, there is no cooking involved, it tastes wonderful, is extremely satisfying and, as a bonus, is very, very good for you.

leaves of 1 baby cos lettuce, washed
200g/7¼ oz baby spinach leaves, washed
2 carrots, peeled and grated
2 beetroots, peeled and grated
100g/3½ oz snow peas, sliced
2 tomatoes, sliced
½ Spanish onion, sliced
1 Lebanese cucumber, sliced
1 avocado, sliced
4 x 185g/6½ oz cans tuna, drained
1 cup crumbled fetta

DRESSING
1 tablespoon olive oil
1 tablespoon white wine vinegar
1 tablespoon lemon juice
sea salt and pepper

To make the dressing, combine olive oil, vinegar, lemon juice and salt and pepper in a cup. Whisk well and set aside.

Place lettuce, spinach, carrot, beetroot, snow peas, tomato, onion, cucumber and avocado in a large mixing bowl and toss with the prepared dressing.

Divide salad between 4 pasta bowls.

Place tuna on top of each salad and arrange feta around the tuna.

SERVES 4

MEDITERRANEAN SALAD

I guess this is a cross between a Greek and a Niçoise salad. You can play around with it as you like. For example, you can replace chickpeas with borlotti beans, or perhaps leave out the parsley and use snow pea sprouts instead.

6 tomatoes, diced
2 Lebanese cucumbers, sliced
½ Spanish onion, finely sliced
1 red capsicum, cut into strips
400g/14¼ oz can chickpeas, rinsed and drained
2 cups flat-leaf parsley leaves
8 anchovy fillets, chopped
16 kalamata olives
8 hard-boiled eggs, quartered

DRESSING
1 tablespoon olive oil
1 tablespoon white wine vinegar
1 tablespoon lemon juice
sea salt and pepper

To make the dressing, combine olive oil, vinegar, lemon juice and salt and pepper in a cup. Whisk well and set aside.

Place tomato, cucumber, onion, capsicum, chickpeas, parsley, anchovies and olives in a mixing bowl and toss with the prepared dressing.

Divide salad between 4 pasta bowls.

Arrange eight egg quarters on top of each salad.

SERVES 4

Mediterranean salad

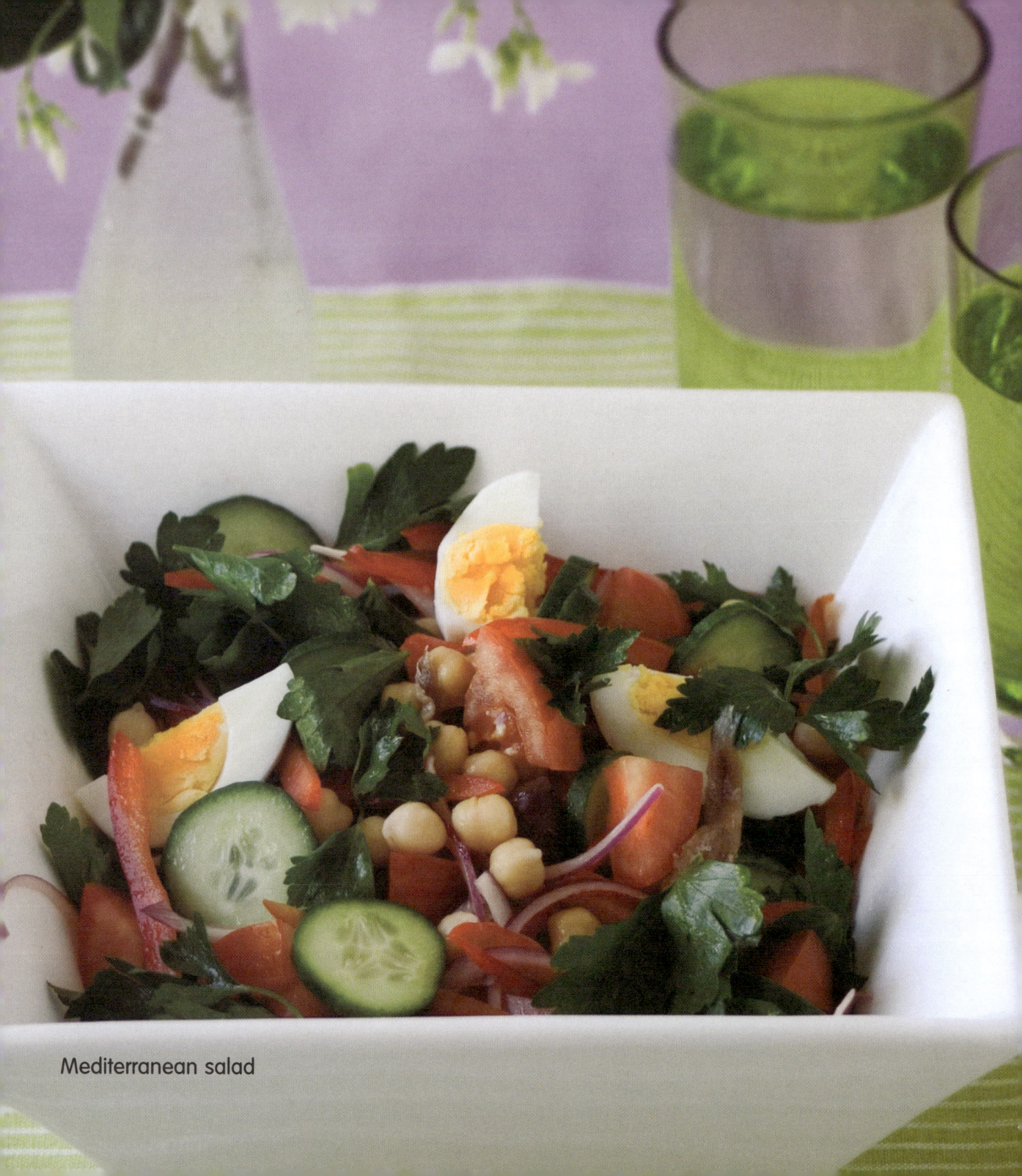

Beans, legumes and pulses

Having spent far too long as the butt of rude jokes, the humble bean has finally come of age. Take baked beans, for instance. Once relegated to the back of the cupboard, they're now being given the royal treatment. However, there are more beans out there than just baked ones—try soya, kidney, cannellini, borlotti, adzuki and broad beans.

Apart from being low in fat and high in fibre (both soluble and insoluble), beans are a great source of protein (particularly when combined with grains like rice and wheat), and contain oligosaccharides (which are great food for good bowel bugs like acidophilus and bifidus) as well as plenty of vitamins and minerals, particularly the B vitamins and iron. Beans also provide phyto (plant) hormones, which may help prevent breast and prostate cancer. And they have a really low glycaemic index, making them an excellent food for losing weight and stabilising blood sugars.

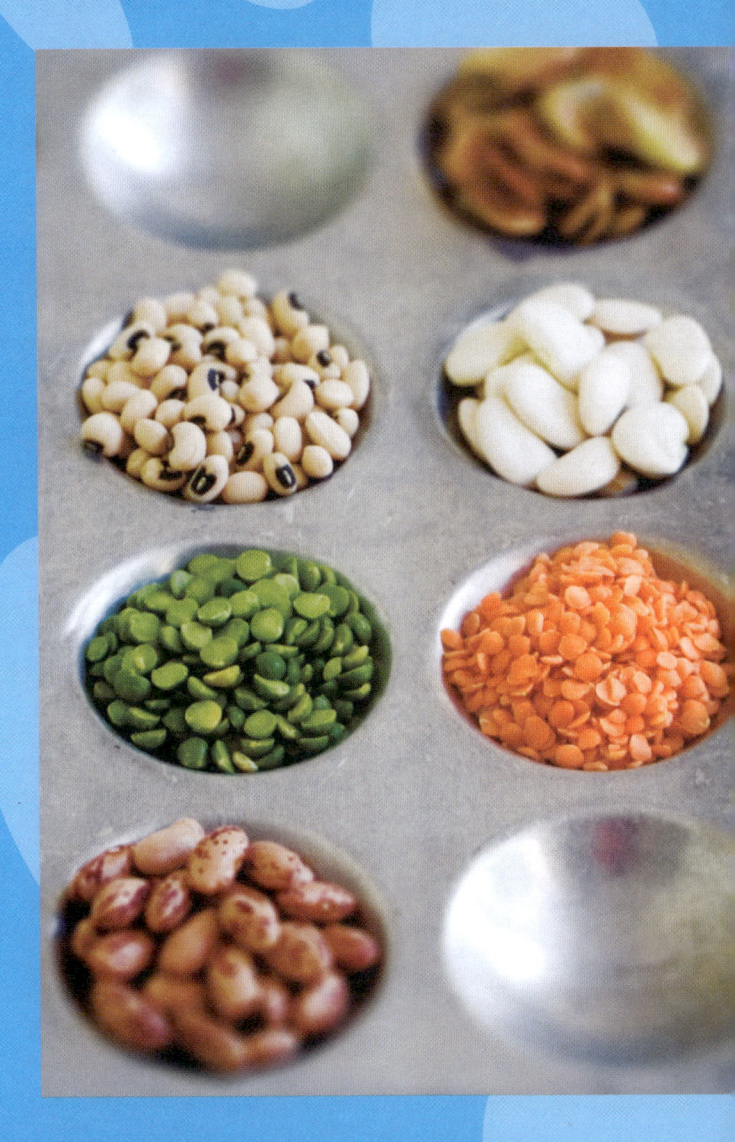

feelgood food

LENTIL SALAD

Don't be put off by having to cook the lentils—they take no time at all. Dried lentils are much tastier than the canned variety.

2 cups dried brown or green lentils
½ cup olive oil
½ cup white wine vinegar
½ cup lemon juice
2 tablespoons finely chopped thyme leaves

TO SERVE

4 cups baby spinach leaves, washed
juice of 1 lemon
4 tomatoes, diced
1 beetroot, peeled and grated
1 cup crumbled feta
sea salt and pepper
extra virgin olive oil, for drizzling

Place lentils and 6 cups of cold water in a large saucepan. Bring to the boil, reduce heat to low and simmer for 5 minutes. Drain lentils and rinse under cold running water. Return to the pan and again cover with 6 cups of cold water. Bring to the boil, reduce heat to low and simmer until lentils are tender (about 15 minutes).

Drain lentils and transfer to a bowl. Mix through olive oil, vinegar, lemon juice and thyme. The dressed lentils will keep in the fridge, covered, for up to 5 days.

To serve, place spinach leaves in a mixing bowl and toss with lemon juice. Portion spinach onto 4 dinner plates.

Toss 2 cups of lentils with tomato and beetroot, and place on spinach leaves.

Arrange feta on the lentils, season with salt and pepper and drizzle with a little extra virgin olive oil.

SERVES 4

OMELETTE WITH FETA & DILL

This is my mother's recipe—she makes a flat omelette, but I like to fold it over. It tastes good either way.

8 eggs
1 cup crumbled feta
½ cup finely chopped dill
sea salt and pepper

Break eggs into a large mixing bowl, and give them a quick whisk.

Add feta, dill and salt and pepper, and whisk.

Spray a large non-stick frypan with a little canola or olive oil cooking spray, and heat pan on medium heat.

Pour beaten egg mixture into the hot pan and cook for about 3 minutes until the edges are cooked and underneath is golden. (At this stage the middle of the omelette will still be wet.)

Lift the omelette on one side with an egg slice and fold it over to form a semicircle. Remove pan from heat and set aside for a few minutes. The middle part of the omelette, which is inside the fold, will cook in its own heat.

Cut omelette into quarters and place each quarter on a dinner plate. Serve with a side salad of mixed leaves and tomatoes.

SERVES 4

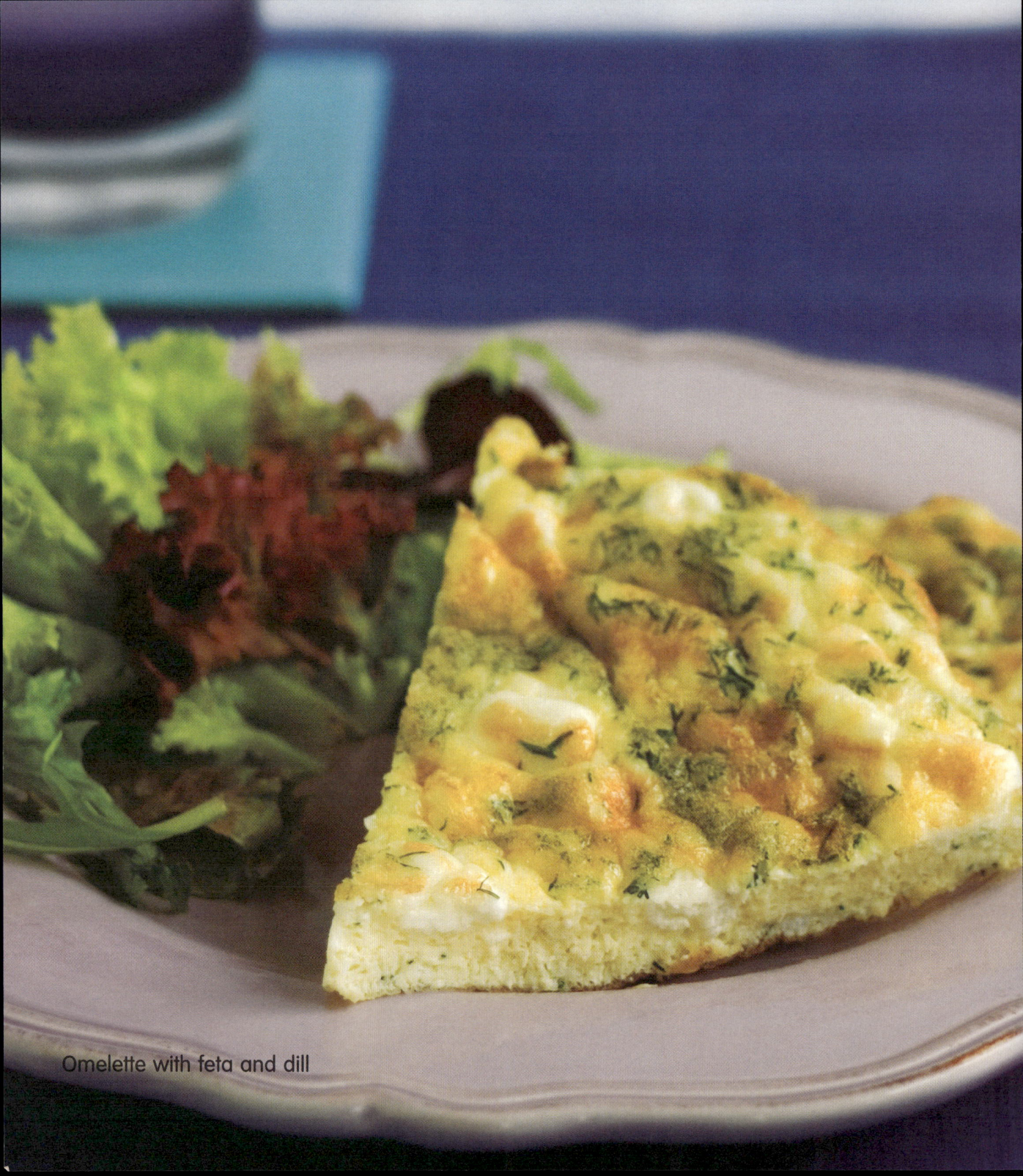

Omelette with feta and dill

Beetroot

Twenty years ago, beetroot came sliced, canned and dressed in vinegar and sugar. Likely sightings were beside potato salad or pressed between a slice of pineapple and fried onions on a hamburger. Nowadays, the dusty-looking beetroot proudly takes its place alongside the other vegetables at your local greengrocer.

Beetroot is a rich source of nutrients. For a start, it's particularly high in antioxidant carotenoids, as well as magnesium, folic acid and fibre. Beetroot plays a starring role in the vegetable juices promoted by Drs Bircher-Benner and Gerson early last century as cleansing tonics beneficial for those with chronic diseases, including cancer. Beetroot has more recently been acclaimed for its liver-cleansing properties. As the liver is our prime detoxifying organ, and helps with, among other things, fat metabolism, including beetroot in your diet makes good sense. Beetroot can be steamed or baked, and raw beetroot can be grated in salads or added to vegetable juices.

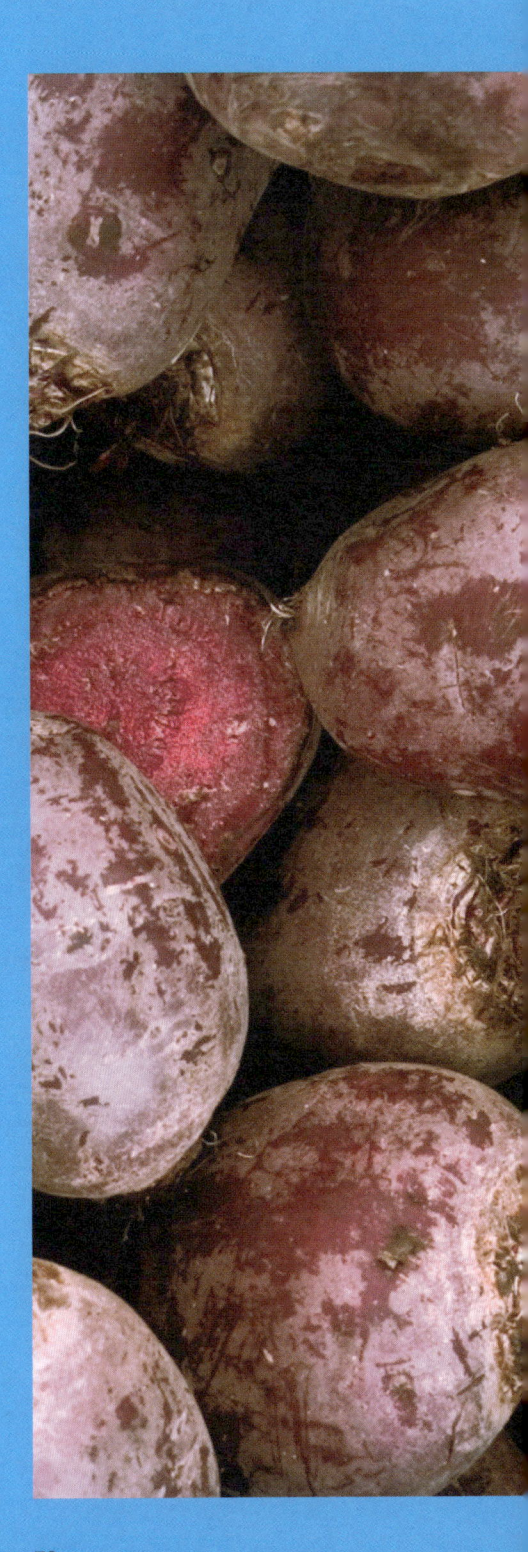

SPANISH OMELETTE

You can make this omelette with just about any leftovers you find in the fridge. It is delicious hot or cold and particularly good with some crusty bread. You don't have to stick to the ingredients I've listed below, but the more variety you have the tastier the omelette.

2 tablespoons olive oil
4 small new potatoes, boiled until tender and diced
4 Roma tomatoes, seeds removed and diced
3 small zucchini, sliced
1 red capsicum, cut into strips
1 baby eggplant, diced
100g/3½oz green beans, cut into quarters
½ Spanish onion, chopped
2 garlic cloves, crushed
½ teaspoon chilli paste or 1 fresh chilli, finely chopped
½ cup chopped thyme leaves
½ cup finely chopped flat-leaf parsley
1 cup pitted black olives, cut into halves
sea salt and pepper
8 eggs, beaten
2 tablespoons freshly grated Parmesan (optional)

Heat oil in a large non-stick frypan on medium heat. Add potato, tomato, zucchini, capsicum, eggplant, beans, onion, garlic and chilli. Stir-fry for 10 minutes.

Stir in thyme, parsley and olives and season to taste.

Pour in eggs, shake the pan a little so the eggs spread evenly over and around the vegetables. Cook for a couple of minutes.

When the bottom of the omelette is cooked, remove the pan from the heat. Sprinkle over a little Parmesan, if you like, and put the pan under a hot grill to finish cooking. Cook for about 2 minutes or until the top is golden.

Turn omelette out onto a plate and cut into quarters.

SERVES 4

BEEF SALAD

You can replace rump steak with leftover cold roast beef for this salad.

500g/1lb 1½ oz rump steak, fat removed
leaves of 1 baby cos lettuce, washed
1 bunch baby rocket, washed
¼ red cabbage, shredded
1 punnet cherry tomatoes, cut into quarters
1 Lebanese cucumber, sliced
1 red capsicum, cut into strips
½ Spanish onion, sliced
½ cup chopped coriander leaves
soy sauce

DRESSING
1 tablespoon olive oil
1 tablespoon white wine vinegar
1 tablespoon lemon juice
sea salt and pepper

To make the dressing, combine olive oil, vinegar, lemon juice and salt and pepper in a cup. Whisk well and set aside until you are ready to use it.

Heat a skillet on a high heat. Cook steak, for three minutes on each side.

Remove steak from pan, set aside to rest.

Place lettuce, rocket, cabbage, tomato, cucumber, capsicum and onion in a large bowl. Toss with the prepared dressing. Portion salad onto 4 dinner plates.

Slice steak thinly across the grain and arrange over each salad. Sprinkle coriander and soy sauce over each salad.

SERVES 4

Beef salad

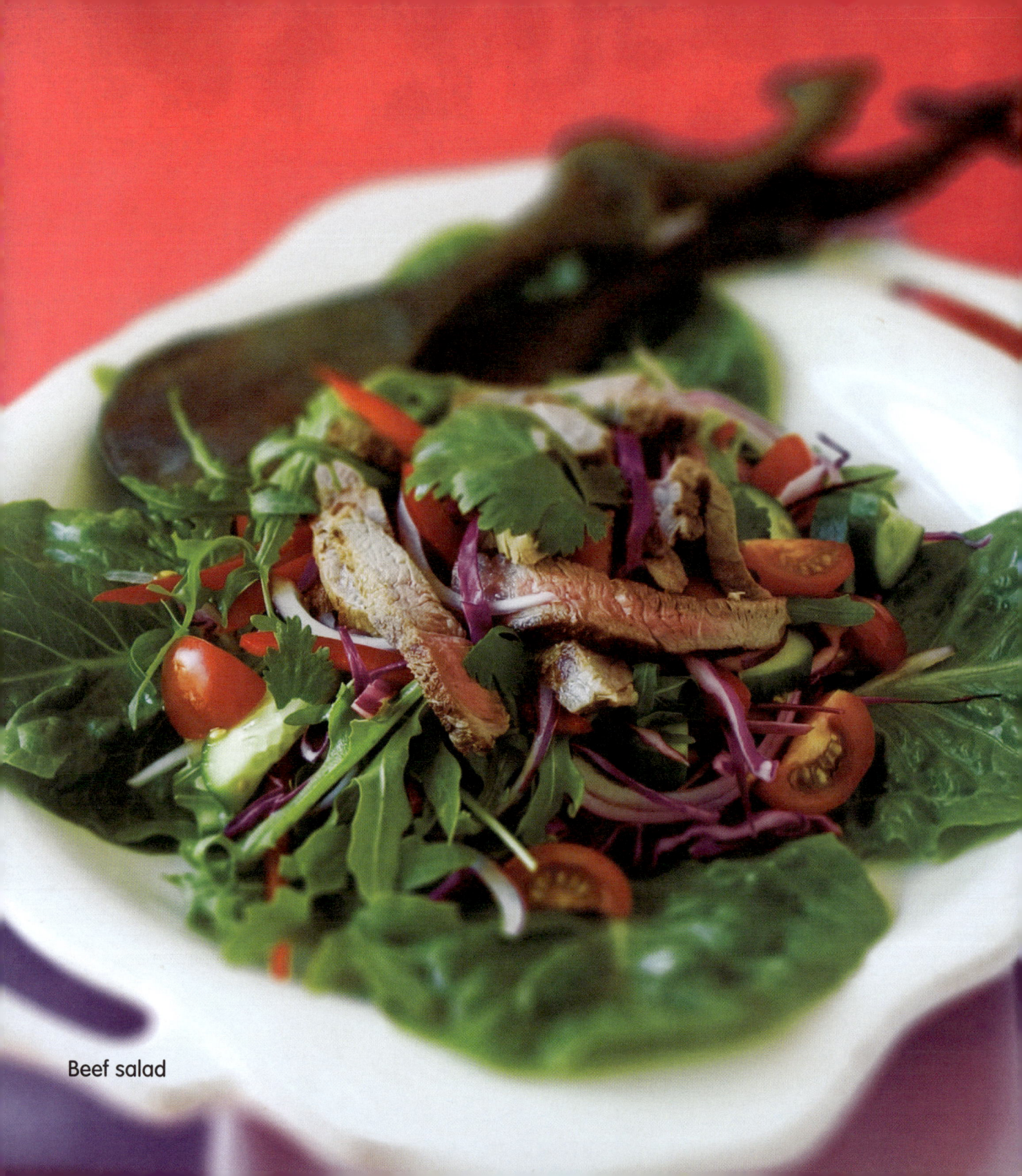

Miso

Miso is a paste made from fermented soya beans. Originating in China in 4BC, miso-making moved to Japan around 800AD where it became an art form and miso assumed mythical status—health, longevity and happiness were assured to all who consume this nutritious, delicious food. To make miso, soya beans (sometimes with the addition of brown rice or barley) are fermented with a special mould, called koji, sea salt and some water. The mash is then stored in cedar vats for 1–3 years. A brown, thick and slightly moist paste results, which tastes like Marmite or Vegemite but with more oomph.

Miso contains all the nutrients of the mother bean, including protein, essential fatty acids and phytonutrients. Also present are calcium and many B vitamins, including B12 (produced by koji mould), which is usually only available from meat and animal products. This mould also produces beneficial substances similar to acidophilus in yoghurt, making it excellent for digestive problems, such as bloating and flatulence. Apart from being jampacked with nutrients, miso is low in calories; though it's high in salt—but if most of your diet is unprocessed, the extra sodium shouldn't pose a problem.

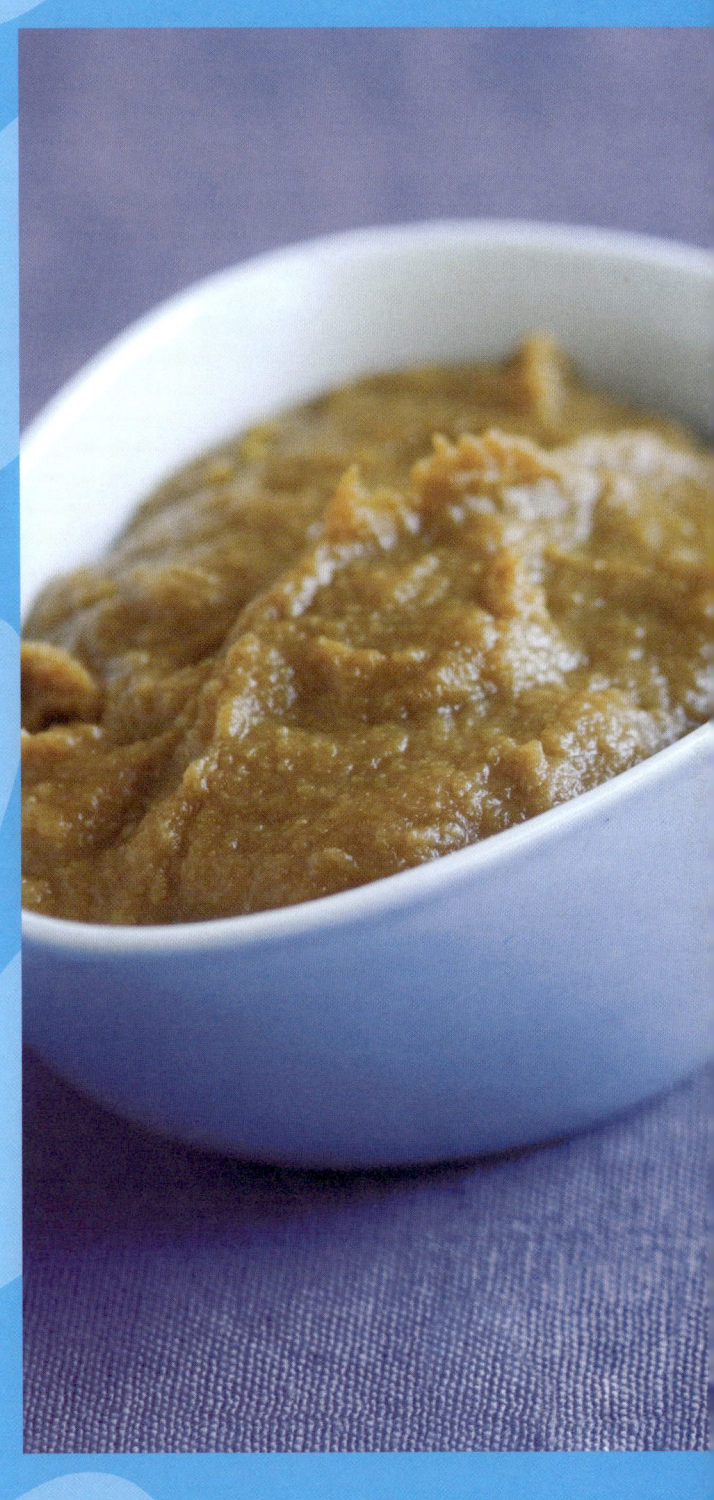

feelgood food

PEA SOUP

I've left out the bacon bones in this recipe because I wanted to keep it vegetarian. However, if you want to add animal protein to the soup, try it with lamb shanks for a change.

3 cups green split peas
2 tablespoons extra virgin olive oil
1 onion, diced
½ bunch thyme, tied with string (so that it can be discarded after the soup is cooked)
2 bay leaves
400g/14½oz can diced Italian tomatoes
6 cups hot water
1 tablespoon miso paste
sea salt and pepper

Put peas in a large sieve and rinse well under hot running water.

Heat oil in a large, heavy-based saucepan. Add onion, thyme and bay leaves and cook for 2 minutes, stirring frequently.

Add tomatoes, split peas and water. Mix well and bring to the boil. Reduce heat and simmer gently for 30 minutes or until the peas and tomatoes have cooked to a pulp.

Discard thyme and bay leaves, stir in miso paste and season to taste. Don't allow the soup to boil after you add miso paste—miso is a live food and boiling will destroy its enzymes, vitamins and probiotics. If soup is too thick, add a little hot water and simmer for a few minutes longer.

SERVES 4

MINESTRONE WITH PESTO

Traditional minestrone uses short pasta, like penne or macaroni. but I haven't included it here because I prefer it without the starch. If you wish to add pasta to the soup, do so after the vegetables are cooked. One cup of penne, spirals, macaroni or similar should be adequate.

2 tablespoons extra virgin olive oil
2 onions, finely diced
2 carrots, diced
3 celery sticks with leaves, finely chopped
2 medium potatoes, peeled and diced
3 zucchini, diced
10 green beans, chopped
¼ cabbage, shredded
400g/14¼ oz can diced Italian tomatoes
1 tablespoon tomato paste
6 cups hot water or vegetable stock
400g/14¼ oz can cannellini beans, drained and rinsed
sea salt and pepper
Pesto (p113)

Heat a large, heavy-based saucepan. Add oil and onion and cook until onion is transparent (about 5 minutes).

Add carrot and celery and cook for 2 minutes.

Add potato, zucchini, green beans, cabbage, tomatoes, tomato paste and water or stock and bring to the boil. Reduce heat to low, cover, and simmer gently for 45 minutes.

Stir in cannellini beans, season to taste, cover and simmer for another 15 minutes.

Serve in soup bowls and place a dollop of pesto on top.

SERVES 4

Minestrone with pesto

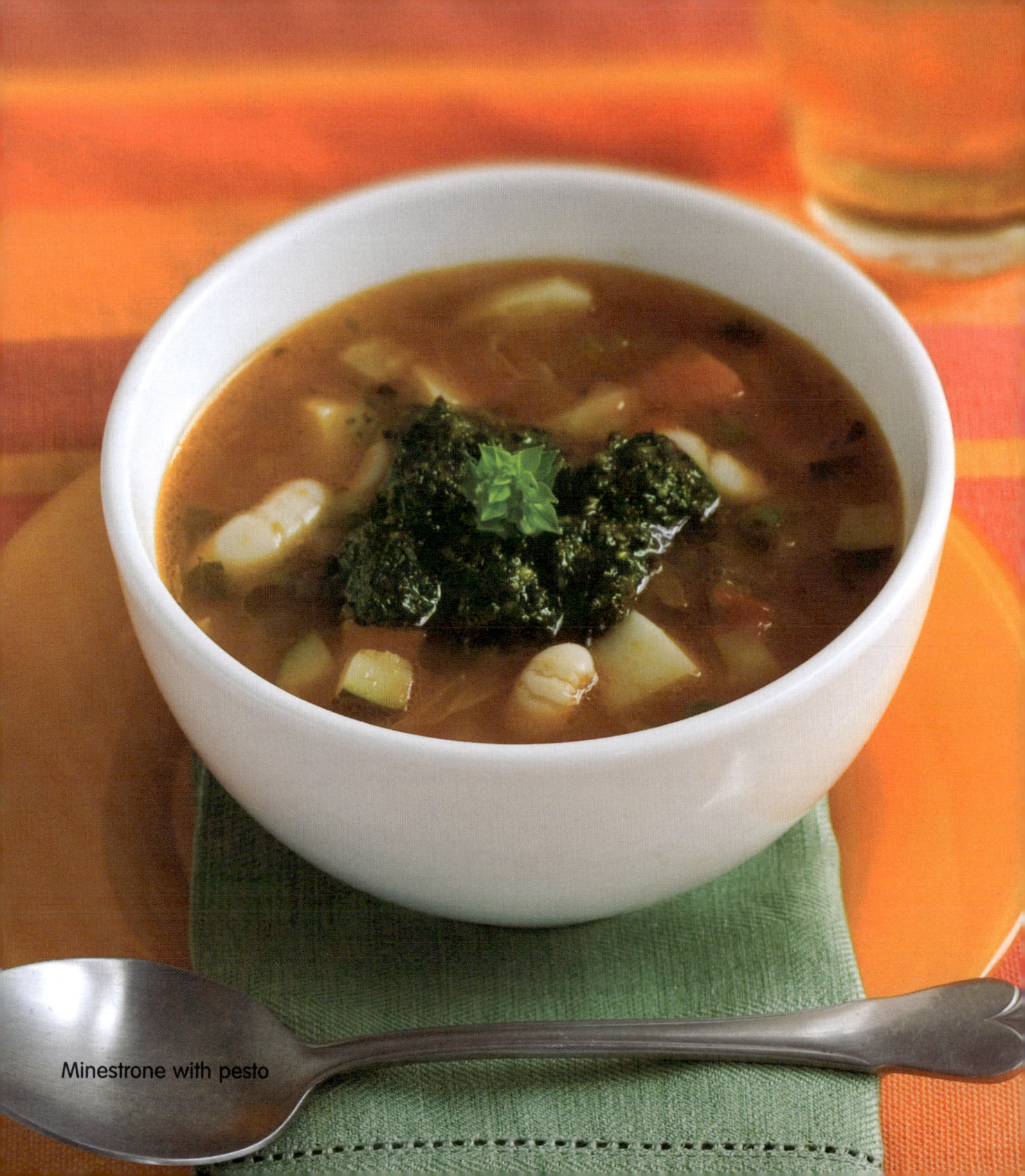

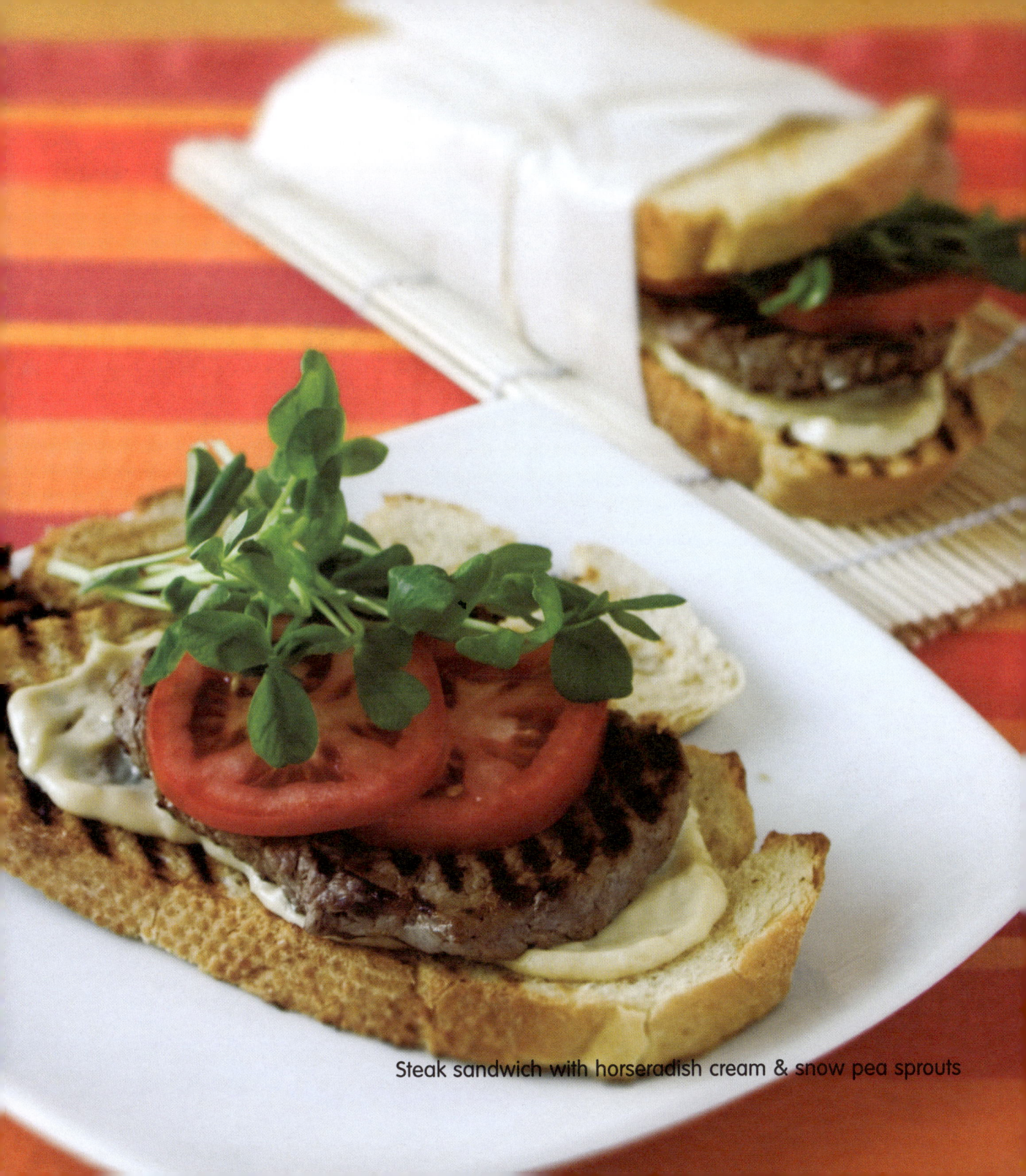

Steak sandwich with horseradish cream & snow pea sprouts

STEAK SANDWICH WITH HORSERADISH CREAM & SNOW PEA SPROUTS

This is always a good lunch when you're feeling a bit run-down and haven't had a good breakfast. Have plenty of paper napkins handy.

4 x 125g/4¼ oz rump steaks, flattened with a mallet
1 tablespoon olive oil
sea salt and pepper
1 tablespoon horseradish cream
8 thick slices wood-fired bread
1 punnet snow pea sprouts
4 Roma tomatoes, sliced

Brush steaks with a little olive oil and rub with salt and pepper.

Cook steaks in a skillet on a high heat for 3 minutes each side.

Spread horseradish cream on 4 slices of the bread.

Place snow pea sprouts on the remaining 4 slices of bread. Arrange slices of tomato and a piece of steak on top.

Close each sandwich with a piece of bread, which has been spread with horseradish cream.

SERVES 4

ZUCCHINI SLICE

If you have a little more time, for variation, make pancakes with this batter. Cook them in a non-stick frypan, but be warned: they can burn easily.

6 zucchini, grated
2 eggs
1 cup crumbled feta
1 cup plain flour
½ cup finely chopped dill
½ cup finely chopped mint leaves
sea salt and pepper

Preheat oven to 180°C/350°F.

Mix zucchini, eggs, feta, flour, dill, mint, and salt and pepper in a mixing bowl. Mix until a thick batter forms.

Transfer zucchini mixture to an oiled baking dish, approximately 28 x 18cm.

Bake in oven until the top of the zucchini mixture turns golden brown (40–45 minutes).

Serve hot or cold with a side salad.

SERVES 4

BROWN RICE & TUNA SALAD

For variation, you can replace tuna with chopped hard-boiled eggs.

2 cups cooked brown rice
4 x 185g/6½ oz cans tuna, drained and flaked
3 tomatoes, diced
1 cup snow peas, sliced
1 cup finely chopped mint and coriander leaves
1 Lebanese cucumber, diced
½ Spanish onion, finely diced
½ cup unsalted, roasted peanuts

DRESSING
1 tablespoon olive oil
1 tablespoon white wine vinegar
2 tablespoons lime or lemon juice
½ teaspoon chilli paste
sea salt and pepper

To make the dressing, combine olive oil, vinegar, lime or lemon juice, chilli paste and salt and pepper in a cup. Whisk well and set aside.

Place rice, tuna, tomato, snow peas, mint, coriander, cucumber, onion and peanuts in a large bowl and mix to combine.

Toss the prepared dressing through the salad.

Serve in 4 pasta bowls.

SERVES 4

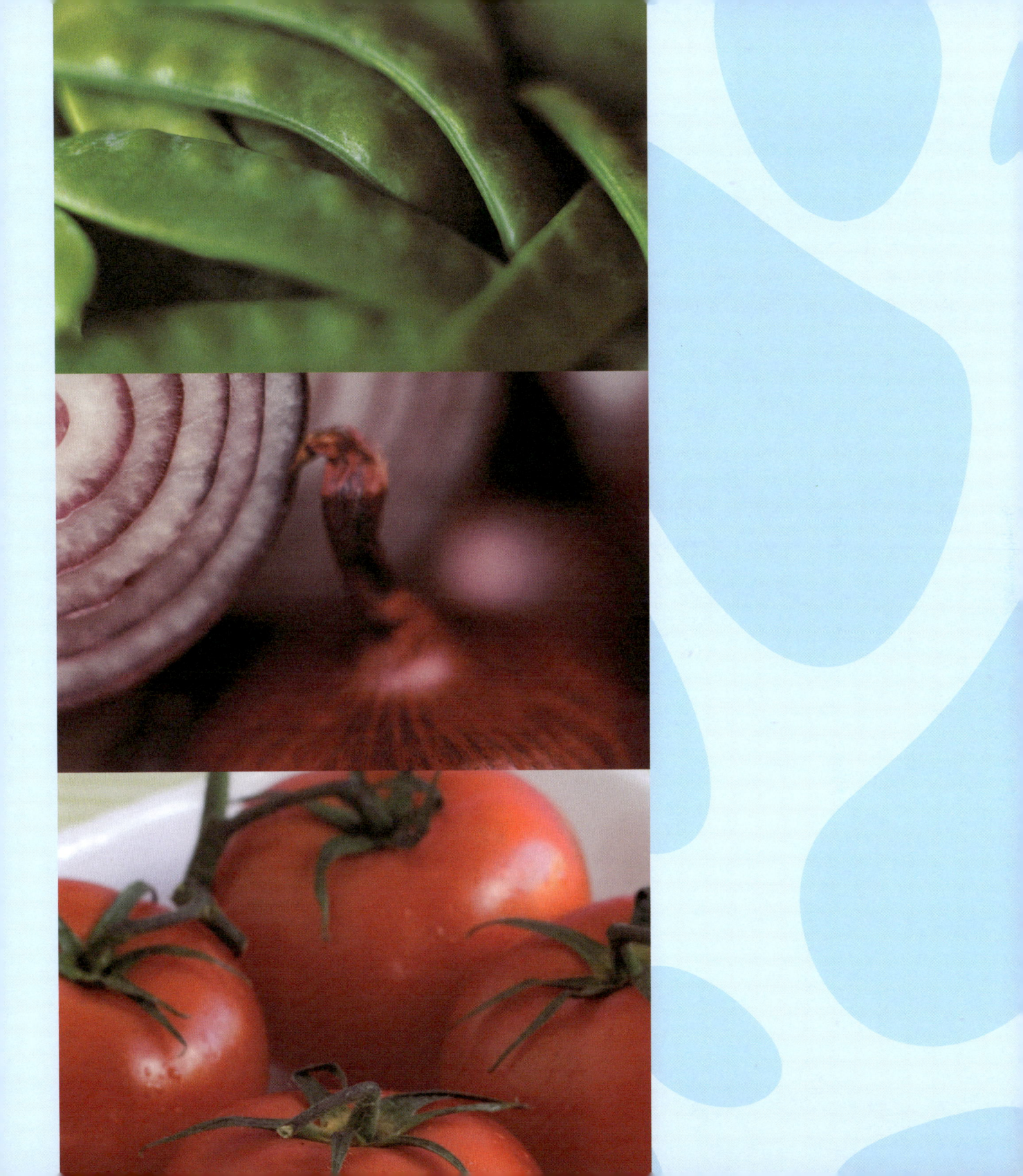

RED LENTIL SOUP

I grew up in a household where legumes featured regularly on the menu. My mother introduced them into our diet from a very early age. I still eat them at least twice a week.

500g/1lb 1½ oz split red lentils
2 tablespoons olive oil
1 onion, finely chopped
1 red chilli, finely chopped
1 large carrot, peeled and diced
2 baby eggplants, diced
1 tablespoon ginger, grated
2 teaspoons ground cumin
400g/14¼ oz can Italian tomatoes, crushed
2 garlic cloves, crushed
6 cups hot water
juice of 1 lemon
½ cup chopped coriander leaves
sea salt and pepper

Place lentils in a sieve, rinse under hot running water and set aside to drain.

Heat oil in a large, heavy-based saucepan. Add onion, chilli, carrot, eggplant, ginger and cumin and cook for about 5 minutes.

Add lentils, tomatoes, garlic and water. Bring to the boil, reduce heat to low and simmer gently until lentils are cooked to a pulp (20–30 minutes).

Add lemon juice and coriander, and season to taste. If the soup is too thick, add a cup of boiling water and simmer for a few more minutes.

SERVES 4

CARROT & GINGER SOUP WITH CORIANDER

If you want to add protein to this soup, stir through some diced tofu just before serving. Or you can purée the tofu with the soup, which will give it an ultra creamy texture.

Ingredients	Method
2 tablespoons olive oil 1 onion, diced 2 tablespoons ginger, grated 1 chilli, deseeded and finely chopped 1kg/2lb 3$\frac{1}{4}$ oz carrots, peeled and sliced 4 cups hot water 400g/14$\frac{1}{4}$ oz can coconut milk 2 tablespoons honey sea salt and pepper 1 cup chopped coriander leaves	Heat oil in a large, heavy-based saucepan. Add onion, ginger and chilli and cook for three minutes or until the onions are transparent. Add carrot, water and coconut milk and bring to the boil. Reduce heat and simmer until carrots are soft (about 25 minutes). Add honey and stir until dissolved. Remove from heat. Purée soup with a hand blender or in batches in an electric blender. Season soup to taste and stir through coriander.

SERVES 4

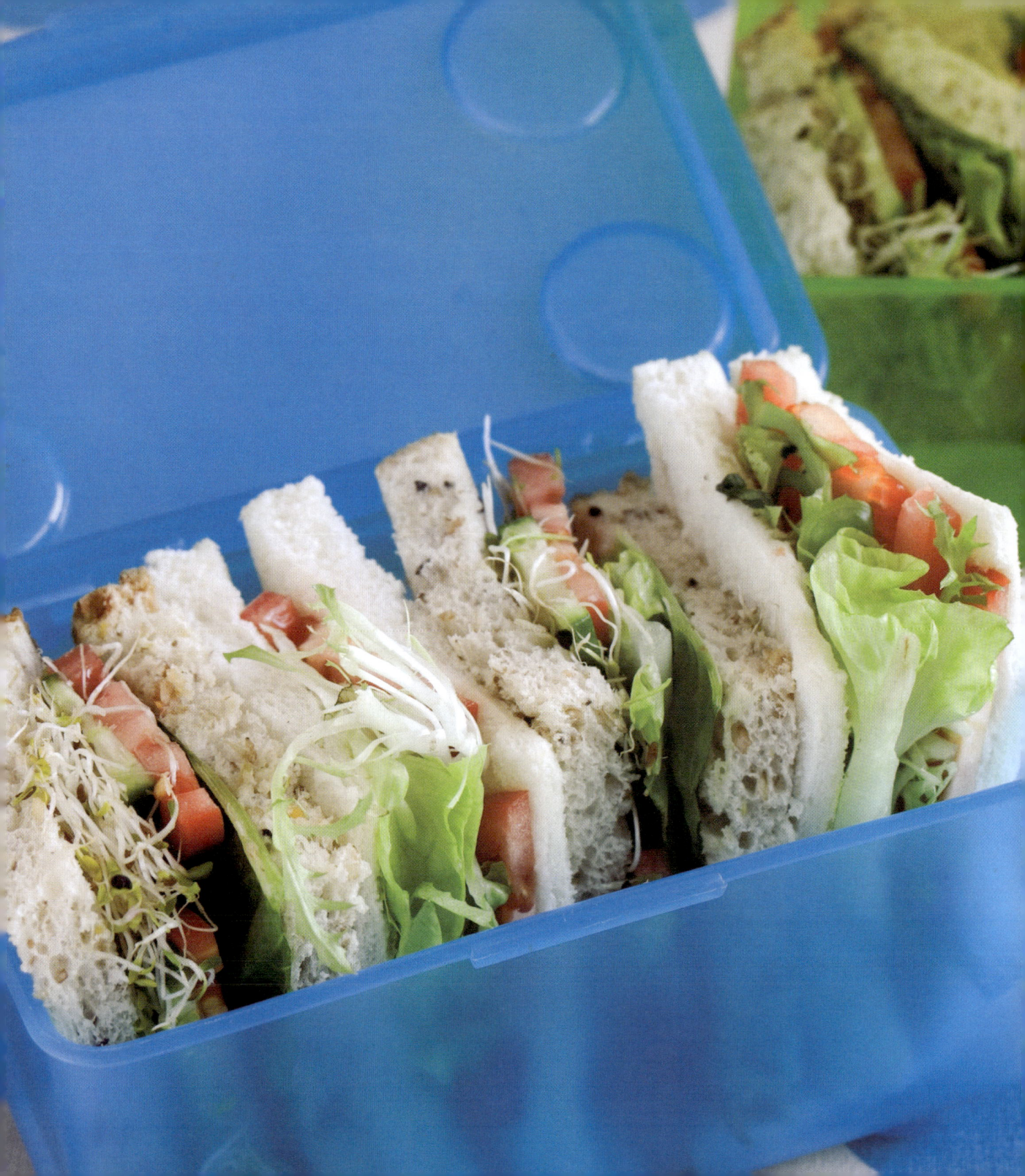

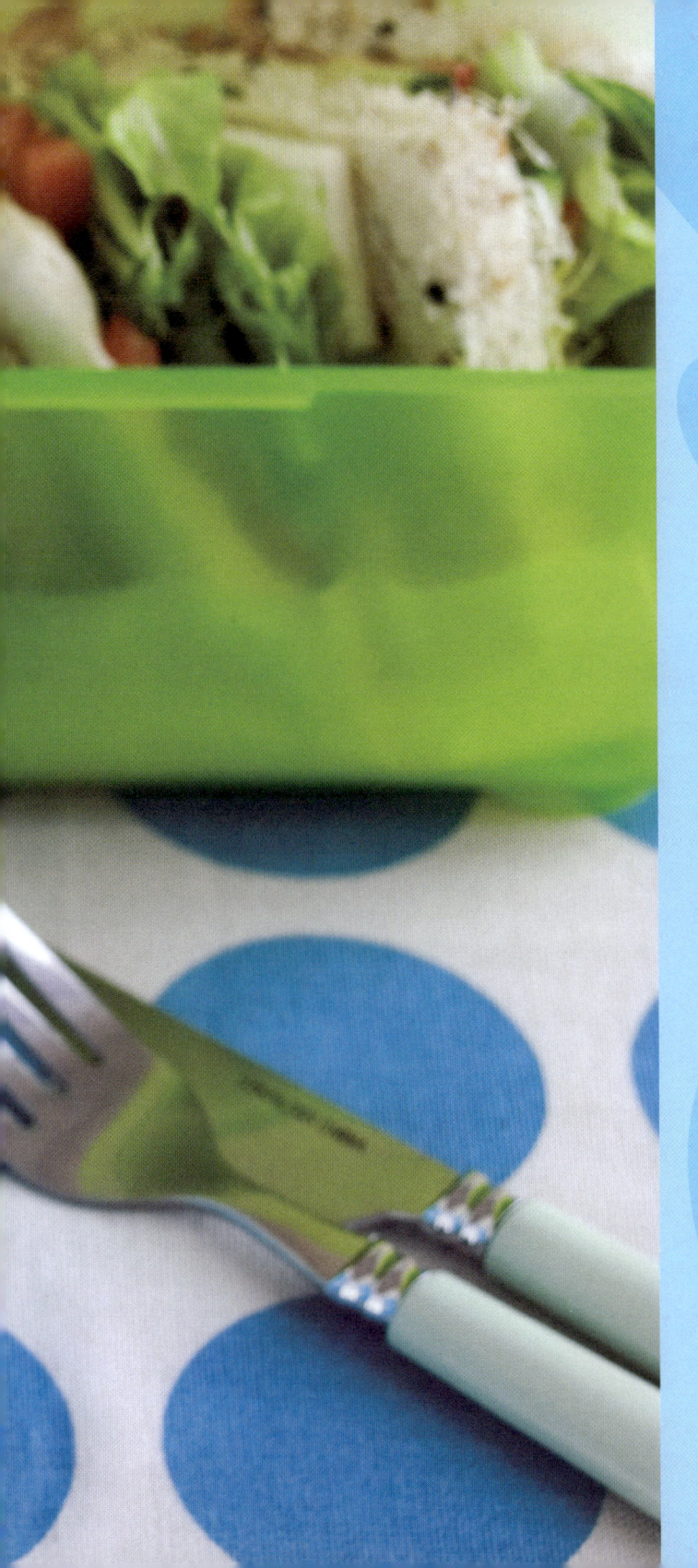

Lunchboxes

How often have you gone to the trouble of preparing lunch for everyone in the morning rush, only to discover in the evening that it wasn't eaten? How often have you asked yourself why you bother at all? I hope the following suggestions will put an end to lunchbox rejection.

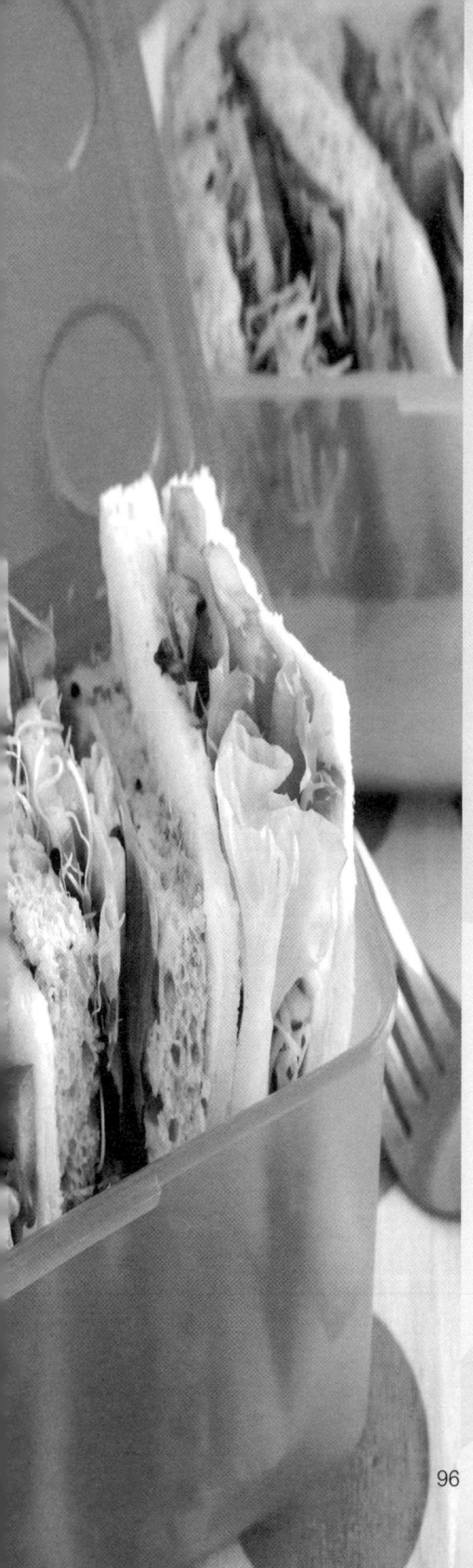

SALADS

Salads are great for lunchboxes, but to be a hit they must be packed well and dressed. To be able to achieve this, you will need:

- large rectangular plastic container with lid—this is for the salad.

- small plastic container to fit inside the large one—this is for the protein component of the salad.

- a disposable/recyclable container with lid (like those tiny containers in which condiments for take away Asian food are stored)—this is for the salad dressing.

Different dressings
Make the following dressings, put them in little containers or jars with lids and store them in the fridge. They will keep for a week.

- Beetroot & yoghurt dip (p161)
- Chickpea & tahini dip (p161)

Make a salad with as many as possible of the following vegetables. Toss well.

- lettuce
- baby spinach leaves
- grated carrot
- tomatoes
- cucumber

- onions
- snow peas
- grated beetroot
- capsicum
- avocado
- baby rocket
- red cabbage

Have different protein components for the salads prepared in advance so you can pack different ones throughout the week. The following are good examples of what you can pack.

- tuna
- hard-boiled eggs
- cold roast beef
- cold grilled chicken
- cold roast lamb
- cold lentils
- canned mixed beans, drained and rinsed
- canned chickpeas, drained and rinsed

Packing tips
Position the various components of the salad into the different containers, storing the two small ones inside the larger. Wrap a paper napkin around a plastic fork, seal it in a small zip-lock plastic bag and store it on top of the salad. Close the container tightly. To save time in the morning, pack the lunch-boxes in the evening and store them in the fridge overnight.

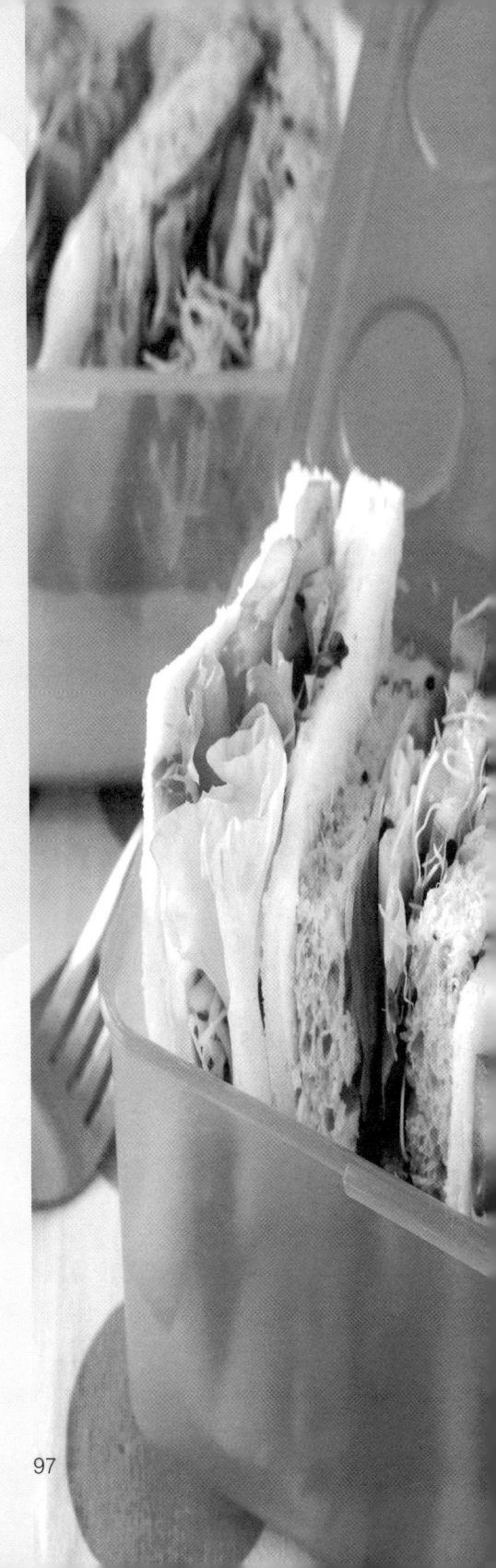

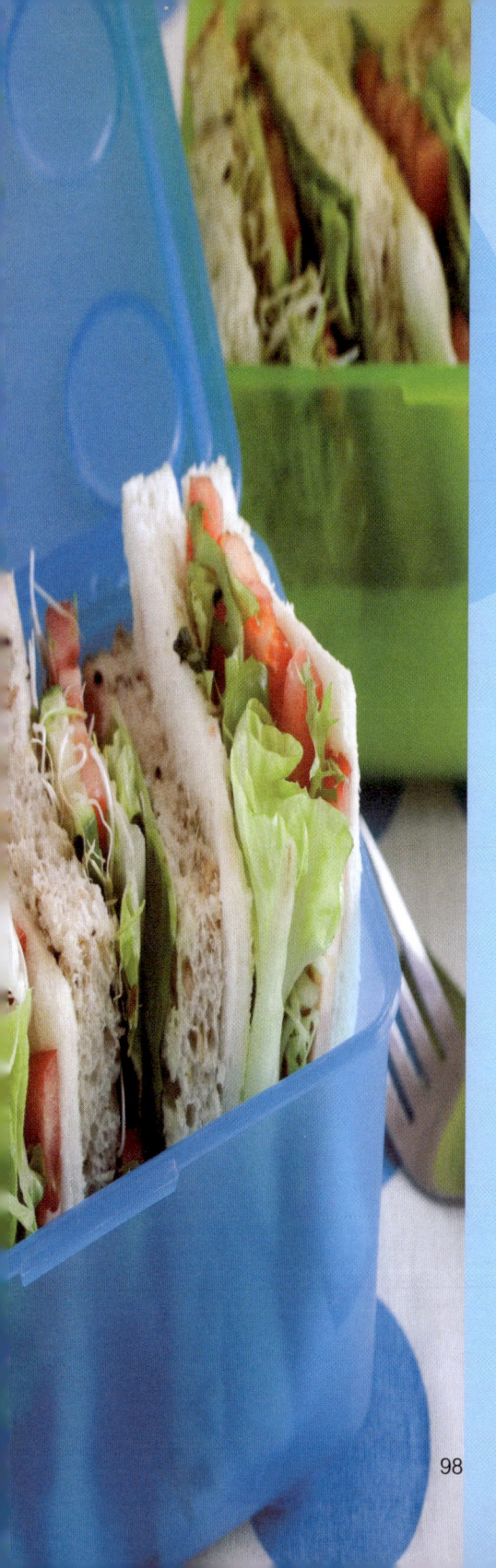

SANDWICHES

While a sandwich is a convenience food at lunch time and can be mouthwatering when made with fresh fillings and crusty breads, it is not always the healthiest option. Many of us consume too much starch each day. Eliminating excess starch from our diets would help prevent obesity and related illnesses and enhance our overall wellbeing. Keep tabs on your family's starch consumption and limit starchy foods to one meal a day, preferably in the mornings.

Now, getting back to sandwiches, they must have healthy and delicious fillings, keep well and not get soggy by lunch time. Here are some suggestions for fillings and bread types:

- use wholemeal, multigrain, sourdough, wholemeal pocket and flat breads.

- use freshly cooked meats—don't be tempted by processed delicatessen meats.

- to stop sandwiches from going soggy, place lettuce, spinach, sprouts or similar greens on the bottom piece of bread, top with other fillings, finish off with another layer of the leafy greens. Close the sandwich with the second piece of bread. This way you will be able to prevent the bread from absorbing moisture.

- for easy handling, cut sandwiches in half, then wrap each half separately. This way they will keep fresher and won't fall apart when unwrapping.

- remember to pack plenty of paper napkins.

Some fillings that will leave you satisfied

- cold roast beef, horseradish cream, lettuce, tomato and grated carrot.

- cold roast lamb, baby spinach leaves, tomato and grated carrot, Chickpea & tahini dip (p161) used as a spread.

- cold chicken, avocado, Spanish onion, tomato and lettuce.

- tasty cheese, tomato, Spanish onion and snow pea sprouts with Olive paste (p161) used as a spread.

- hard-boiled eggs, tomato, Spanish onion, cucumber, capsicum and baby spinach leaves.

- cottage cheese, broccoli spouts, grated carrot, avocado and tomato, Olive paste (p161) used as a spread.

- tuna (well drained), lettuce, tomato, Spanish onion, grated carrot and capsicum.

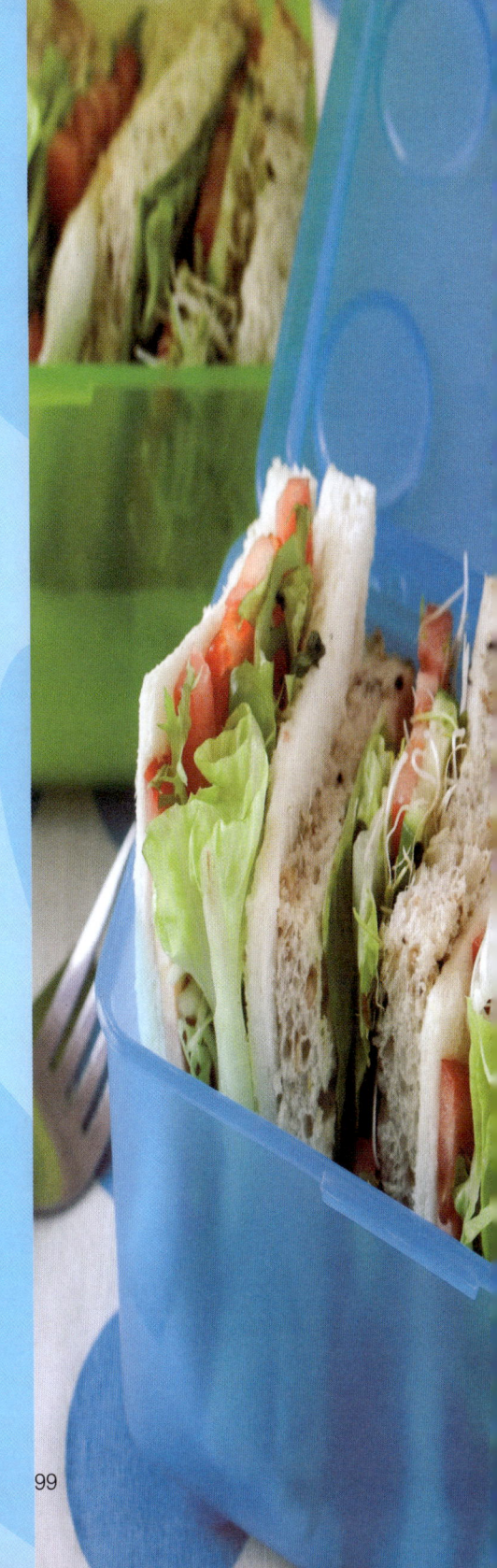

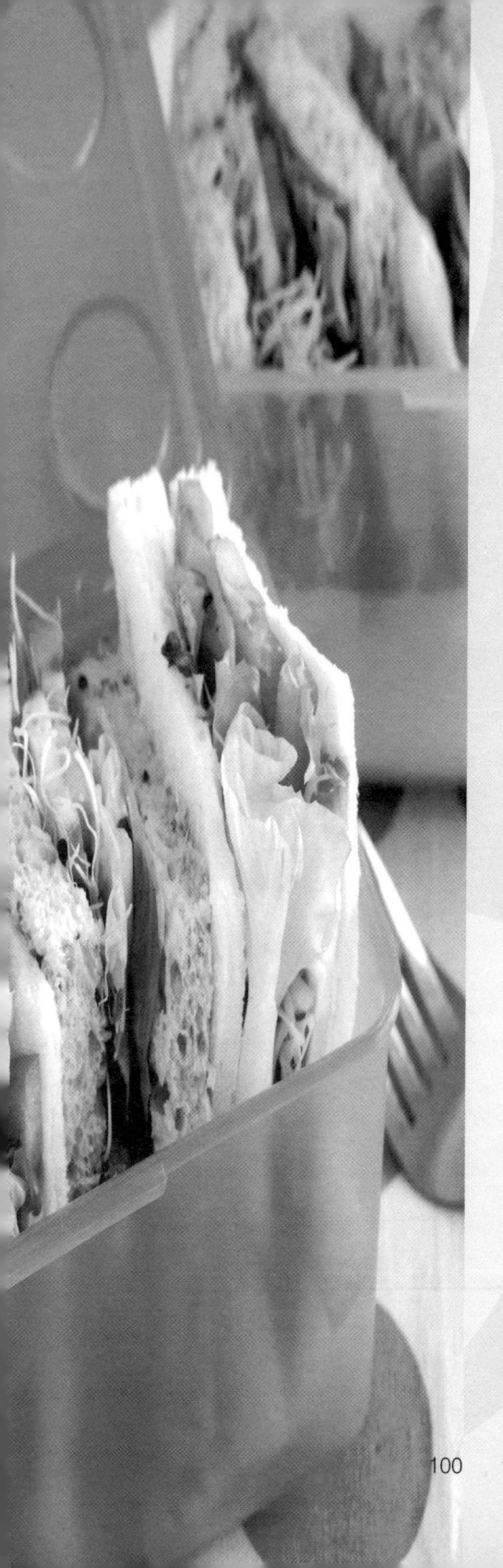

LEFTOVERS

Leftovers are ideal for lunchboxes and take just a little time to pack. Pack them in the same way as you'd pack salads. Use a large container with a lid and a smaller one to fit into it, positioned to one side. Don't forget to pack a dressing for the accompanying salad.

Here are some suggestions:

- Zucchini slice (p89) with a tomato, Spanish onion and parsley salad.

- Spanish omelette (p80) with a green salad.

- Potato & herb salad (p108) with tuna. Toss the tuna through this salad rather than packing it on the side.

- Green beans, pesto & roast tomatoes (p113) with tuna.

- Penne with tuna, olives & capers (p124). This pasta is great hot or cold. Pack a green salad on the side.

SOUPS

Soups are excellent for lunchboxes too, especially on cold winter days. You can heat any leftover soup and pack it into a small thermos. Remember to add some protein to the soup if it doesn't contain any. For example, you can add 100g of diced tofu to tomato or pumpkin soup. Similarly, you can stir through some miso paste for added protein.

Try these:

- Minestrone with pesto (p85)
- Pea soup (p84)
- Red lentil soup (p92)
- Carrot & ginger soup with coriander (p93)

SNACKS

While prepackaged snack foods are convenient, most are high in sugar, salt, colourings and fat. For example, low-fat fruit yoghurt sounds like a good snack choice, right? Actually, not really. Look at the nutrition information list on the container and you'll find that these yoghurts have a very high sugar content. The same is true of most commercial snack foods.

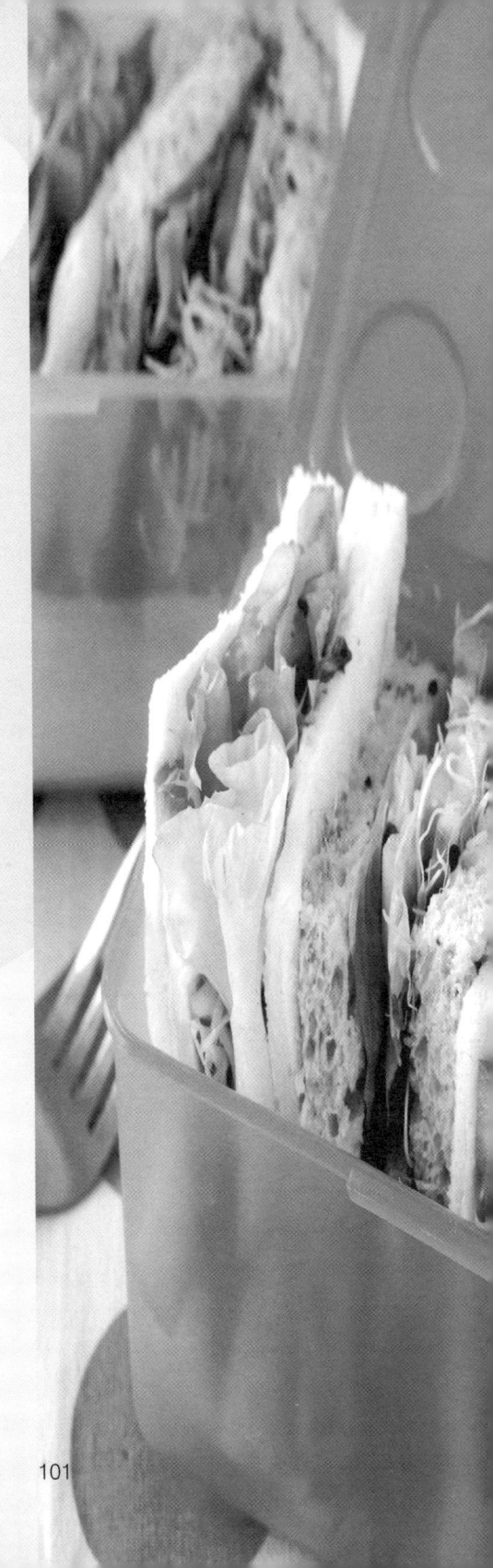

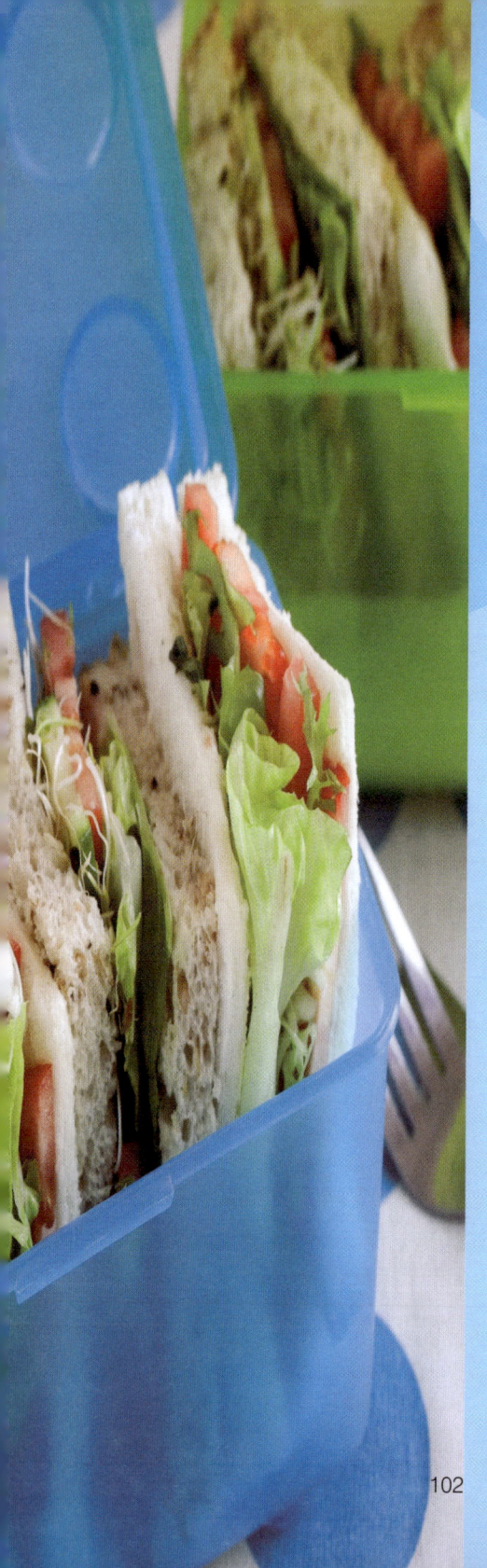

Here is a list of healthy snacks you can add to lunch-boxes.

- Pumpkin & pepita muffins (p158).

- Chocolate & raspberry muffins (p167).

- Apple & blueberry muffins (p166).

- Oat & sunflower-seed cookies (p162).

- Rice paper rolls (p163).

- Dried fruit and nuts. Commercially prepacked snack food portions of these are fine—they don't contain any additives.

- Fresh fruit—on it's own or with natural yoghurt.

- Chickpea & tahini dip (p161). Pack this into a little container (like a salad dressing container) witht some pita bread.

- Beetroot & yoghurt dip (p161). Serve it the same way as the Chickpea & tahini dip.

- Eggplant & tahini dip (p159). Serve it the same way as other dips.

DRINKS

Don't forget to include a bottle of water—and don't be tempted to put in sports drinks instead. I believe it is better to encourage your family and children to drink water regularly and to limit their intake of sports drinks and soft drinks in general. These products can contain a lot of sugar and on a daily basis the average person simply doesn't need them.

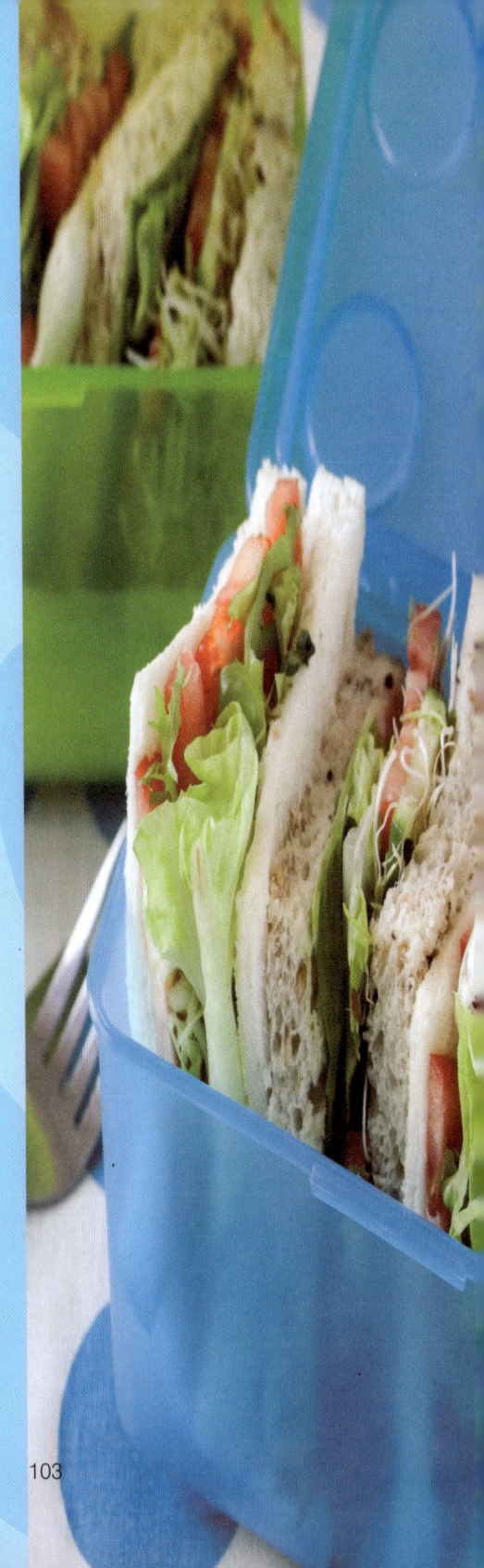

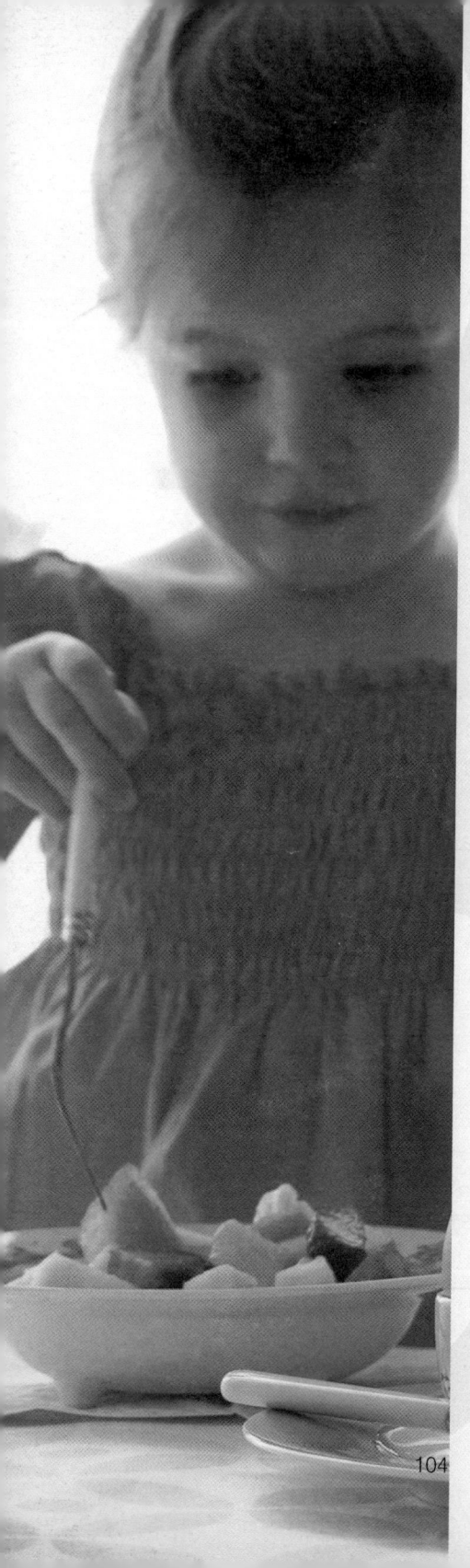

Childzone

Tips for taming fussy eaters

Don't be conned by cute packaging
Those cute packages of cheese and bickies or teeny-weeny chocolates in their own little packs are crammed full of calories. Snacking outside breakfast, morning and afternoon tea, lunch and dinner shouldn't be encouraged, though there is such a thing as wholesome snacks (see pp158–168).

Be firm but fair
Fussy eaters are particularly prone to snacking. It's a hard habit to break, but a little tough love can go a long way. You will feel like a meany (and be told you're one, too), but stick to your guns—no child has yet starved by being deprived of a doughnut.

Waterworld
While adults can be tempted into drinking water with visions of a peach-like complexion, children are less convinced, prefering soft drinks, cordial or flavoured milk. As a treat these are fine, but not as a given. Water is a fine beverage. Also, try not to give drinks before meals—this will fill up children making them less inclined to eat their meal and more inclined to snack.

Family ties
Whenever possible, try to have all the family eat meals together, particularly dinner, even though we spend our adult lives trying to be anything but normal, normality is what children crave. Let them eat what they like when they turn 18.

Smorgasbord
Fussy eaters tend to turn their noses up at what is served on their plate. If you serve the meal on a large plate in the centre of the table and allow each person to serve themselves (or be helped if required), then each person can choose what they wish. What is served on the table is the only thing on offer, so if your little one decides to eat only the mashed potato, that's it until tomorrow morning. Rest assured, their culinary repertoire will soon expand.

Familiarity breeds desire
Introduce new foods regularly to avert a pattern of fussy eating. If a child hasn't seen or eaten a particular food by the time they are seven, they are less likely to try anything new. For little children, new food can be bewildering. Imagine confronting an oyster for the very first time! But if the rest of the family is hoeing into this 'new' food with obvious relish, your child will want some of the action. So keep adding new food to the menu at regular intervals.

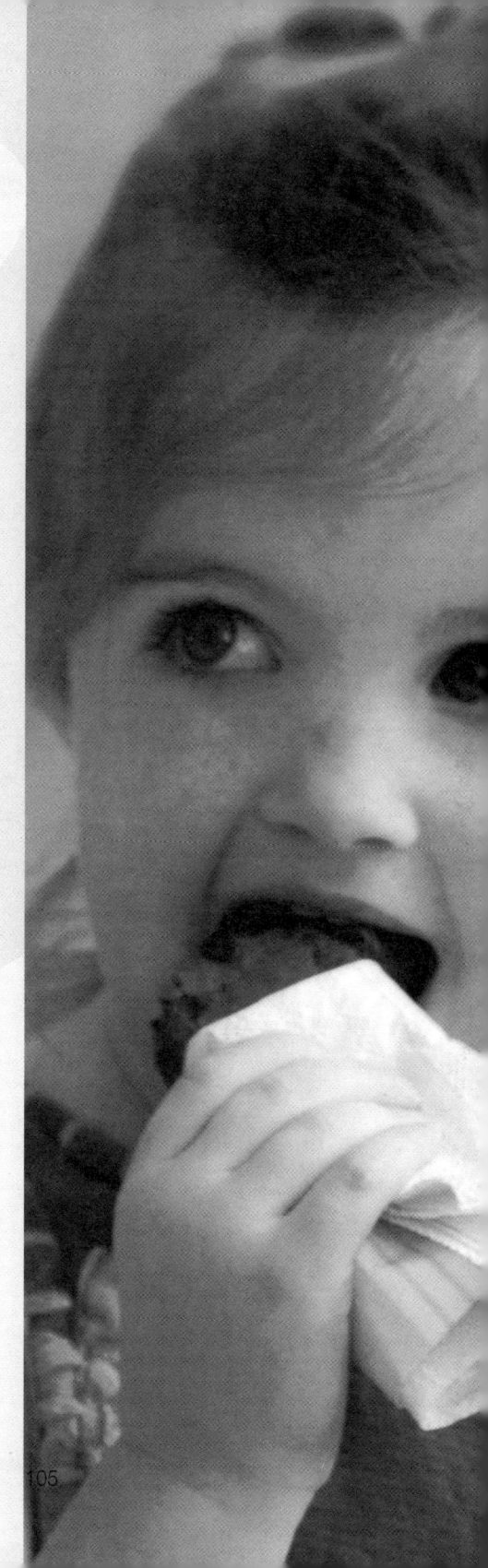

feelgood food

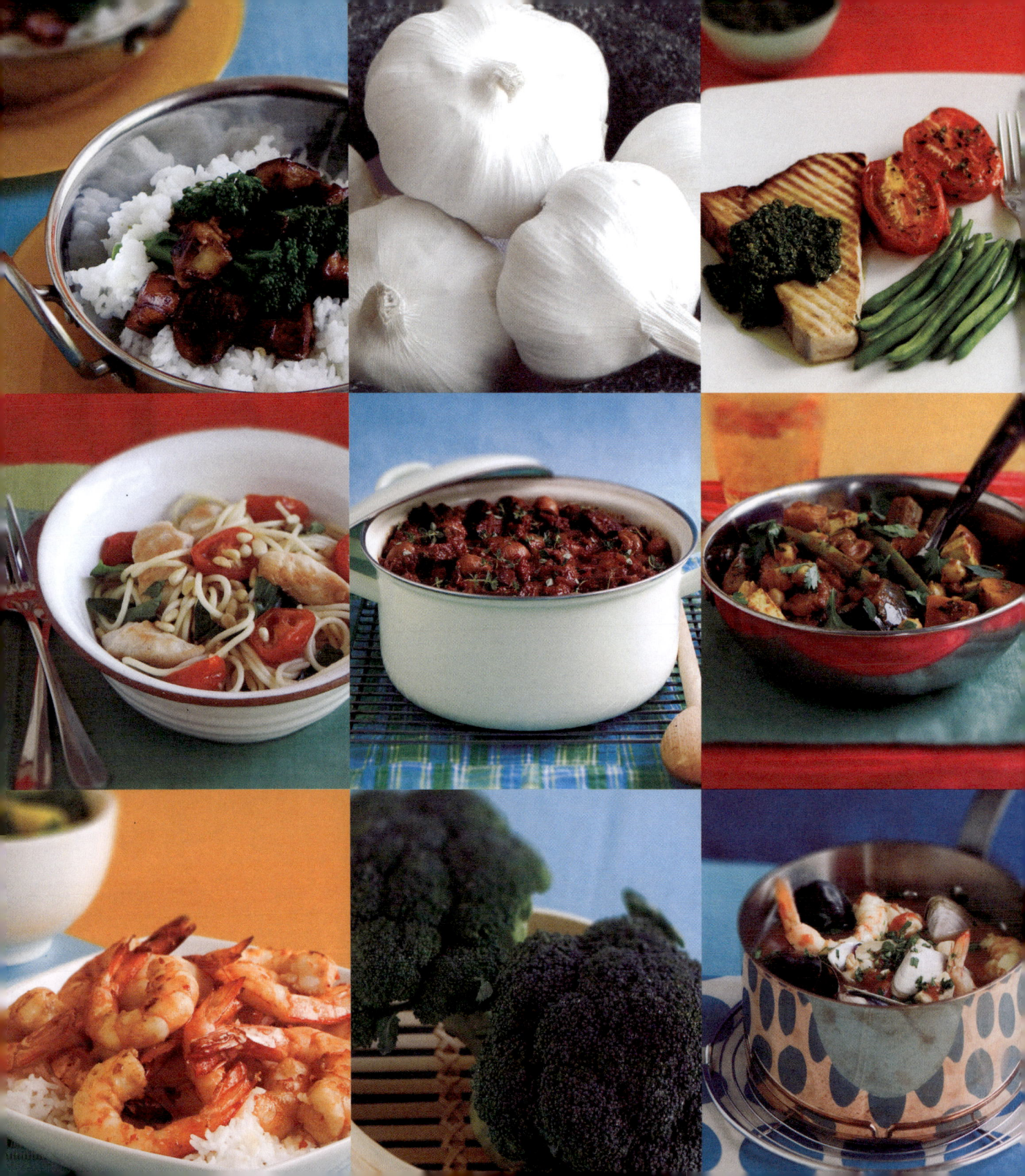

Dinner

Dinner time should and can be a quality and eagerly anticipated time for families—a time for trading tales of the day at the dining table while enjoying delicious, nutritional food. Before you sit down, take the phone off the hook and switch off the television. If you have a young child or children, aim to dine at a time when they are most hungry, and encourage their involvement in the meal's preparation. Most importantly, decide well in advance what's on offer for dinner, and make sure everyone eats the same meal. Though it won't happen overnight, your good eating habits will inevitably rub off on your children. Plus you'll be amazed at the time (and money) you'll save if you all eat the same food. Remember, if you're firm with your family and serve them well-balanced meals, you're setting them on the right path for the rest of their lives.

FLATHEAD FILLETS WITH POTATO & HERB SALAD

In my experience, this dish has always been popular with little ones. They'd even eat the herbs—and come back for more!

POTATO & HERB SALAD
10 waxy potatoes, diced
1/2 cup finely chopped parsley
1/2 cup finely chopped mint leaves
1/2 cup spring onions, sliced
1 cup kalamata olives
2 tablespoons olive oil
2 tablespoons white wine vinegar
sea salt and pepper

600g/1lb 5 1/4 oz flathead fillets, boned and skinned
a little extra olive oil for the fish fillets
squeeze of lemon juice

To make the salad, cook potatoes in salted boiling water until just tender (about 15 minutes). Toss potatoes with parsley, mint, spring onions, olives, oil and vinegar, and season to taste.

Arrange the potato salad on 4 dinner plates and set aside.

Lightly brush fish fillets on each side with the olive oil.

Cook fish fillets under a hot grill for 2 minutes each side. Squeeze lemon juice over them before removing from the grill tray.

Arrange fish fillets on the potato salad and adjust the seasoning if necessary.

SERVES 4

HONEY & SOY CHICKEN WITH RICE

In my Kids' Kitchen days this dish was a big hit in child-care centres. Later, we used the same recipe for frozen, prepackaged meals for school canteens.

3 tablespoons soy sauce
3 tablespoons lemon juice
2 tablespoons honey
6cm/2½ in piece of ginger, grated
2 garlic cloves, crushed
2 teaspoons sesame oil
freshly ground black pepper
1 small red chilli, chopped (optional)
500g/1lb 1½ oz chicken thigh fillets, diced
jasmine rice, to serve

Mix soy sauce, lemon juice, honey, ginger, garlic, sesame oil, pepper and chilli, if using, in a glass, plastic or ceramic bowl (don't use a metal bowl). Add chicken and mix well. Cover with plastic wrap and place in the fridge for at least 1 hour. Stir after half an hour so the marinade evenly covers the chicken.

Heat a large stir-fry pan, add chicken and marinade and stir-fry over high heat for about 5 minutes.

Serve with jasmine rice and green vegetables.

SERVES 4

Honey & soy chicken with rice

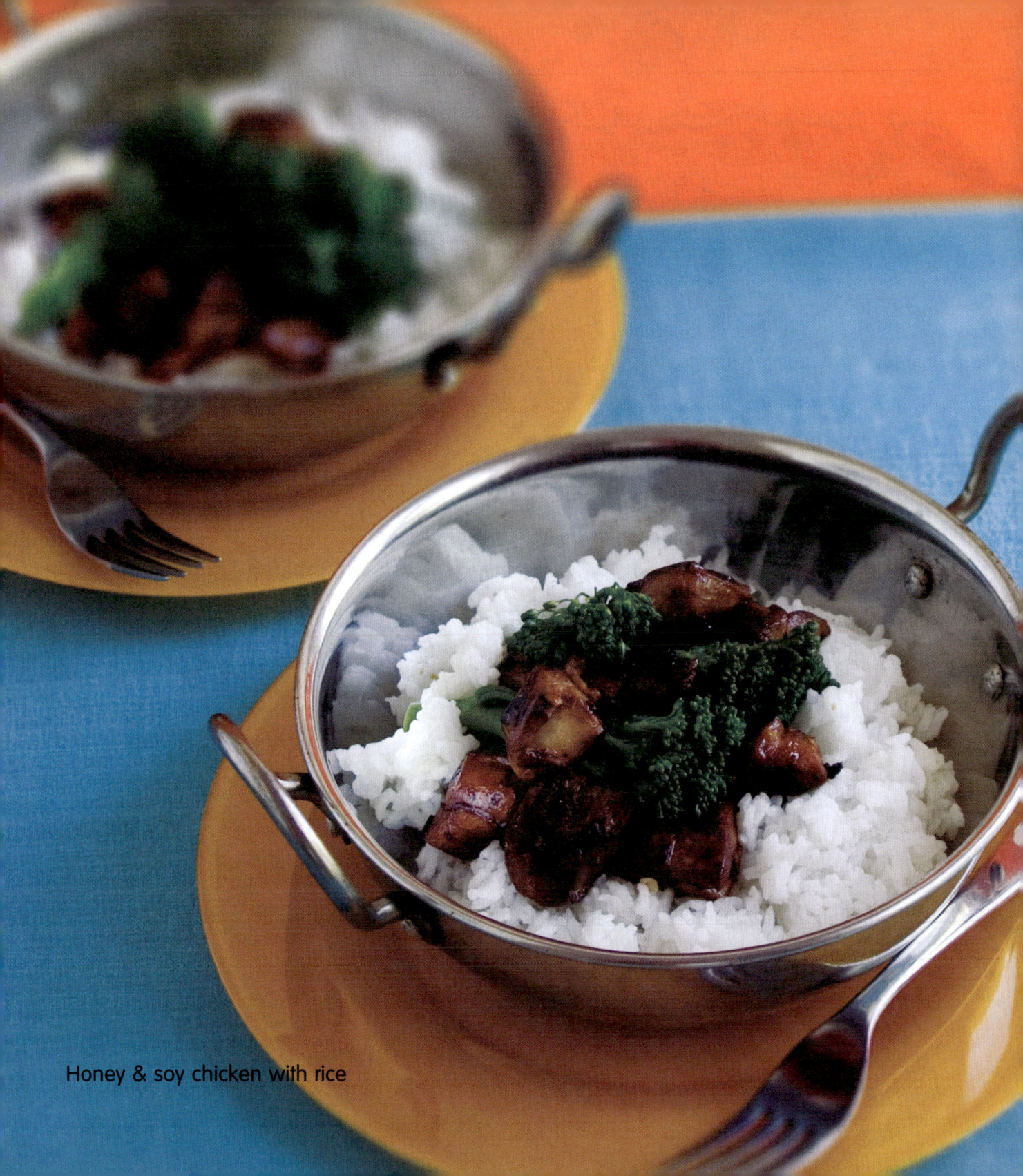

Garlic

From as early as 2000 BC, in Egypt and China, garlic flavoured cuisine and cured ills. In modern times, this powerful bulb's efficacy in preventing and treating heart disease is well documented. Countries such as Italy and Spain, where large quantities of garlic are eaten, boast a low rate of death from heart attacks. When garlic is crushed, the vital compound allicin is released, which helps rid cholesterol from the body, thus protecting against heart and arterial disease. Garlic can also help bronchitis, sore throats, sinus problems, catarrh, asthma, cystitis and other urinary infections, constipation, diarrhoea and stomach upsets—and it can invigorate digestion by stimulating the secretion of enzymes and bile, thus improving general health and vitality. And garlic's benefits don't end there. This super food is believed to have cancer-protective properties, help ward off infection, combat poisoning and even cure athlete's foot—in fact, Roman centurions wedged fresh garlic between their toes to prevent fungal infections. No kitchen should ever be without a head of garlic.

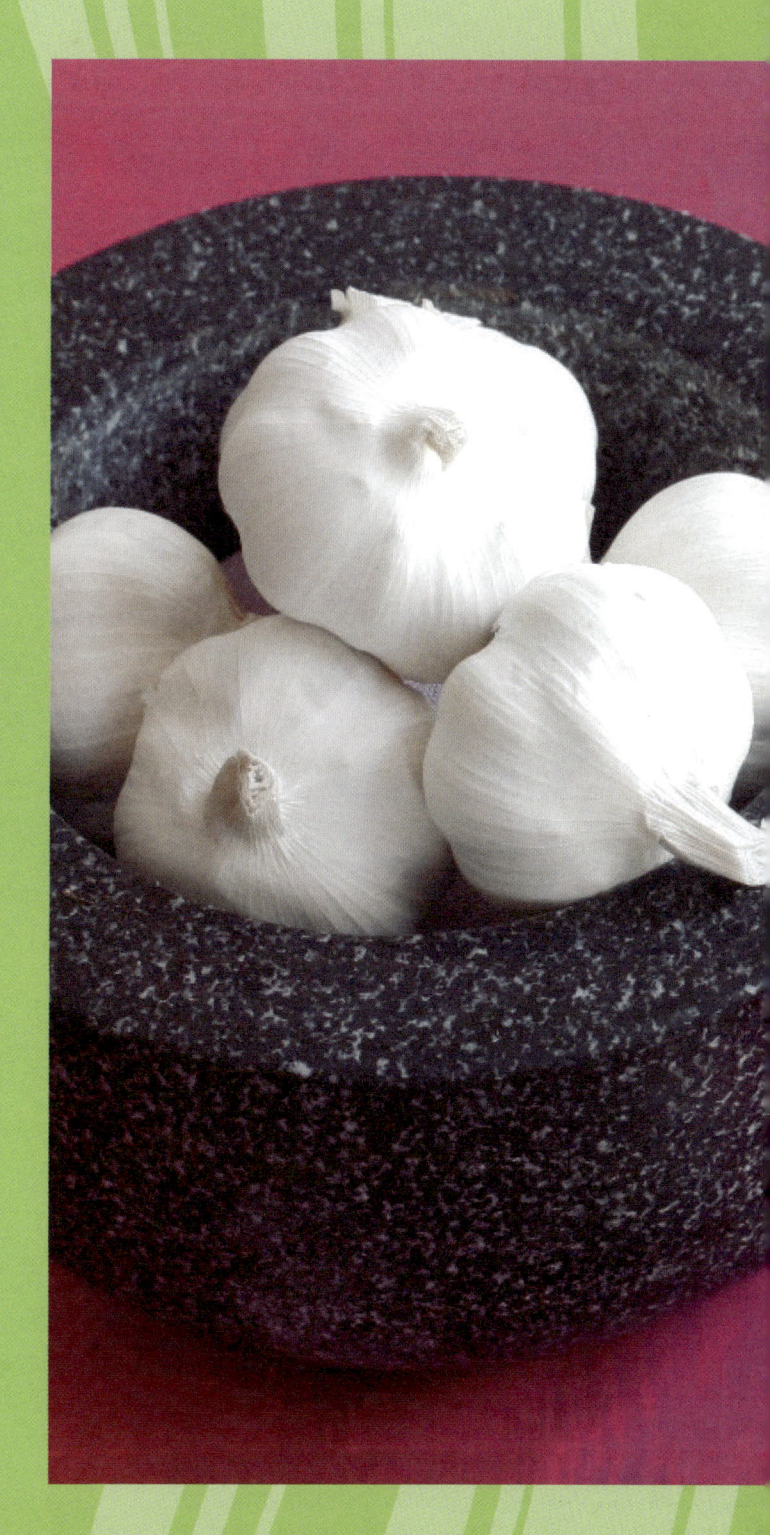

MOROCCAN LAMB WITH COUSCOUS

This isn't an authentic recipe, but it's a pretty good imitation. You can use chicken instead of lamb, if you prefer.

1 tablespoon olive oil
1 onion, finely diced
1 tablespoon grated ginger
2 cinnamon sticks
2 teaspoons ground cumin
2 teaspoons ground turmeric
2 teaspoons ground cardamom
500g/1lb 1½ oz diced lamb, fat removed
2 garlic cloves, diced finely
2 teaspoons harissa or 1 teaspoon chilli powder and 1 teaspoon paprika
400g/14¼ oz can diced Italian tomatoes
sea salt and pepper
½ cup hot water
juice of 1 lemon
½ bunch of coriander, finely chopped
couscous

Heat oil in a heavy-based saucepan. Add onion, ginger, cinnamon, cumin, turmeric and cardamom. Cook for 5 minutes on medium heat or until onion is transparent.

Add lamb to the pan and brown on all sides.

Add garlic and harissa (or chilli and paprika) and stir. Add tomatoes, salt and pepper and hot water, and bring to the boil. Reduce heat to low, cover with lid, and simmer gently for 30 minutes. Don't rush the cooking process—the lamb should be melt-in-the-mouth tender. Continue to simmer gently for another 15 minutes if the lamb is not tender enough. (Remove the cinamon sticks before serving).

Add lemon juice and coriander. Serve with couscous prepared according to the instructions on the packet.

SERVES 4

MARLIN WITH GREEN BEANS, PESTO & ROAST TOMATOES

Kids usually eat vegetables if they have other flavours such as garlic, salt and soy sauce added to them. Pesto is a good choice for flavouring vegetables. You can replace the marlin in this recipe with any firm-fleshed fish.

4 x 200g/7¼ oz marlin steaks
juice of 1 lemon mixed with
1 tablespoon of olive oil
400g/14¼ oz green beans, topped and tailed
4 teaspoons pesto (see below)
sea salt and pepper

ROAST TOMATOES
4 firm, ripe Roma tomatoes, cut in half lengthways
¼ cup olive oil
sea salt and pepper
1 tablespoon finely chopped thyme or oregano

PESTO
2 cups basil leaves
2 garlic cloves, crushed
sea salt and pepper
¼ cup pine nuts, toasted
½ cup olive oil
¼ cup good-quality Parmesan, grated

To make the roast tomatoes, preheat oven to 180°C/350°F. Place tomatoes, cut side up, on a baking tray and sprinkle with oil, salt and pepper and thyme or oregano. Place in the oven and roast for 35–45 minutes or until tomatoes are soft but not falling apart. Set aside. (The cooled tomatoes will keep in the fridge, covered, for up to 5 days).

To make the pesto, place basil, garlic, salt, pepper and pine nuts in a food processor and whizz until basil and pine nuts are finely chopped. While the motor is running, pour ¼ cup of olive oil down the chute in a steady thin stream. Stop the machine and scrape down the sides. Add Parmesan and whizz for a few more seconds. Transfer pesto to an airtight container, pour over the remaining olive oil. The extra oil will rest on top and preserve the pesto. Cover and refrigerate. The pesto will keep in the fridge for 2 weeks, as long as the top of the sauce is always covered with a layer of oil.

Brush marlin steaks with lemon juice and oil mixture.

Heat a skillet on medium high, add marlin steaks and cook for 2 minutes. Brush with remaining lemon juice and oil mixture, turn and continue cooking for 2 minutes. Be careful not to overcook the fish—as soon as the flesh turns white, remove from the heat.

Microwave or steam the beans, toss with 4 teaspoons of the pesto and divide between 4 dinner plates.

Place a marlin steak next to the beans and season to taste. Serve with roast tomato halves.

SERVES 4

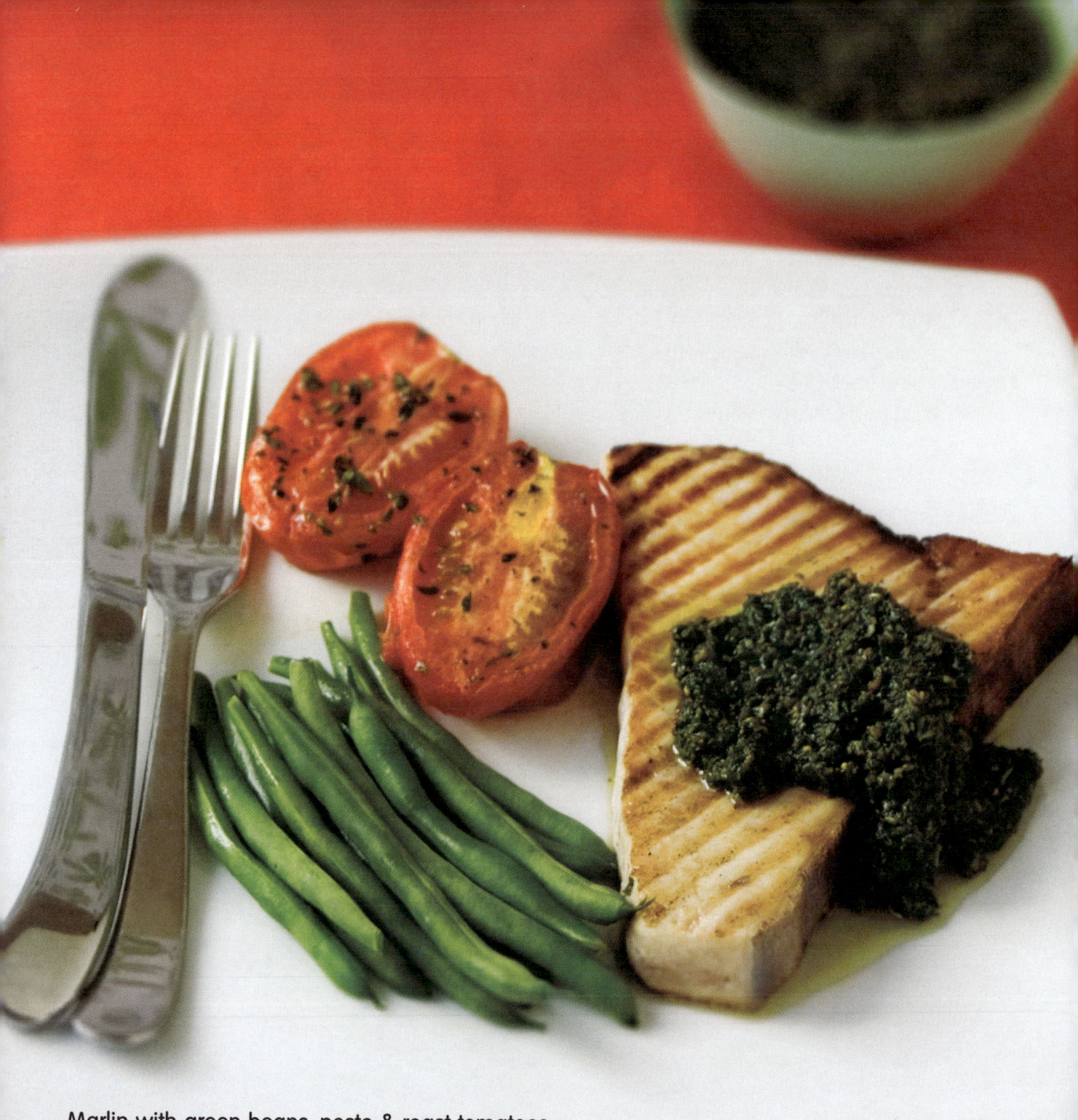

Marlin with green beans, pesto & roast tomatoes

Iron

Iron-deficiency anaemia heads the list as our most common nutritional concern in Australia. Red blood cells need iron to carry oxygen around the body; less iron means less oxygen, which means you feel extremely tired. In addition to fatigue, symptoms of iron deficiency may include recurring infections, irritability, poor concentration, pale skin and sensitivity to the cold.

There are two kinds of iron in the diet: haem iron, found in animal food ('haem' as in haemoglobin), and non-haem iron, found in vegetables and legumes. Haem iron is more readily absorbed than non-haem iron, which is why vegetarians need to watch their iron levels. Vitamin C increases iron absorption of both haem and non-haem iron.

Iron-rich food include lamb, beef, chicken, pork, fish (especially salmon and tuna), eggs, dried fruit (especially peaches, apricots, raisins, dates and figs), molasses, parsley, walnuts, leafy green vegetables (spinach and Asian greens), leeks, lentils, kidney beans, sesame seeds, tofu, pumpkin, watercress, cherries, mulberries, raspberries, strawberries, broccoli and cocoa.

Tea, coffee, cola and some herbal teas can inhibit iron absorption. If you are iron deficient, avoid drinking these for half an hour before meals and one hour after.

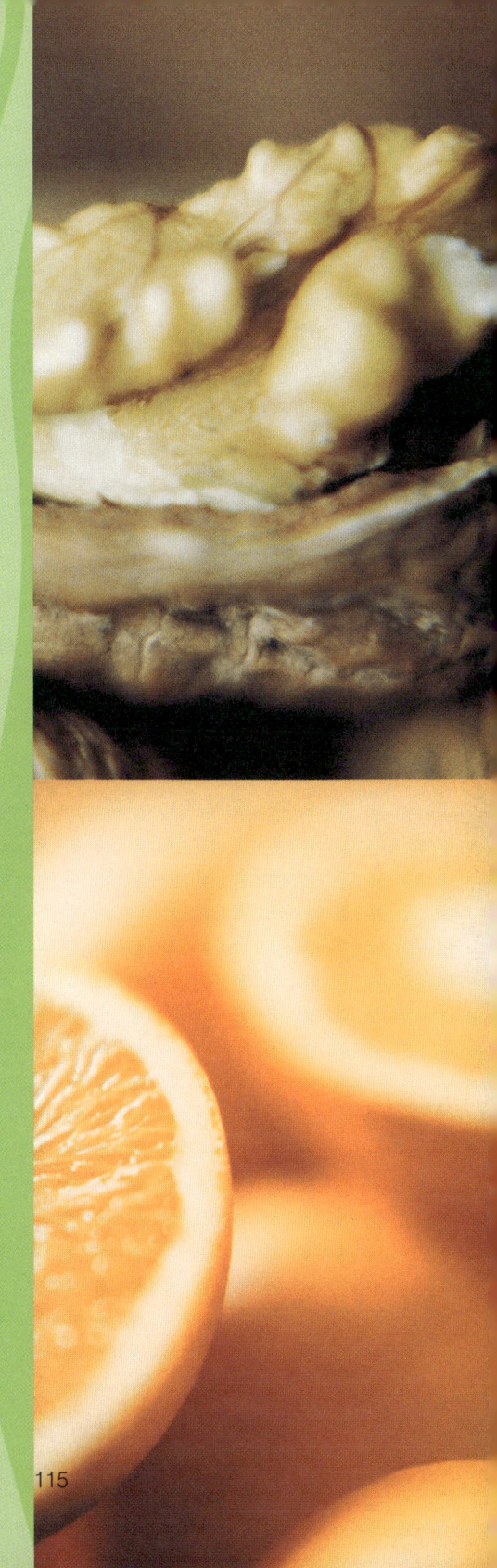

feelgood food

ROAST LAMB WITH ROOT VEGETABLES

This method of cooking without liquid may seem unconventional, but as long as the roasting tin is covered tightly with foil, the meat stays moist. The onion and thyme, which are discarded after cooking, flavour the meat.

1.5kg/3 lb 4½ oz shoulder of lamb on the bone
1 onion, cut in half
½ bunch of thyme
2 medium potatoes, unpeeled and cut into eighths
2 sweet potatoes, unpeeled and cut into slices
1 large carrot, peeled, cut in half lengthways and quartered
1 x 500g/1 lb 1½ oz piece of pumpkin, unpeeled, cut into wedges then cut into slices
1 Spanish onion, peeled and cut into eighths
6 garlic cloves, unpeeled and root ends trimmed
1 tablespoon olive oil
sea salt and pepper
1 tablespoon finely chopped thyme leaves

Preheat oven to 200°C/400°F.

Place lamb, onion and bunch of thyme in a roasting tin. Cover the tin tightly with foil, so steam doesn't escape while roasting. Bake for 1½–2 hours or until the lamb is cooked well and falls off the bone.

Place potatoes, carrot, pumpkin, onion and garlic in another roasting tin. Sprinkle over olive oil, salt and pepper and chopped thyme. Toss well using your hands. Place in the oven 1 hour after you put in the lamb. The vegetables will take 1 hour to cook.

Remove lamb from the oven and set aside to rest for 15 minutes. Discard the onion and thyme and slice the meat. Serve with the roasted vegetables.

SERVES 4

SPAGHETTI WITH CHICKEN, CHERRY TOMATOES, BASIL & PINE NUTS

Although I urge people to eat less starch, I don't think including a couple of pasta recipes is overdoing it.

½ cup pine nuts
500g/1lb 1½ oz thin spaghetti
2 tablespoons olive oil
500g/1lb 1½ oz chicken tenderloins, cut in half
1 punnet cherry tomatoes, cut in half
2 garlic cloves, crushed
sea salt and pepper
1 cup shredded basil leaves
½ cup good-quality Parmesan, shaved

Place pine nuts in a non-stick frypan and toast on medium heat—shake the pan every so often so that they don't burn. Set aside to cool. (If you toast more pine nuts than you need, store them in an airtight container in the fridge).

Cook spaghetti in plenty of rapidly boiling salted water until *al dente*. Drain and set aside.

Heat a stir-fry pan, add oil and chicken, and stir-fry until chicken starts to turn golden. Add tomatoes and garlic and cook until tomatoes are soft (about 3 minutes).

Add pine nuts and season to taste.

Add spaghetti and toss to combine.

Toss through basil and serve immediately, topped with shaved Parmesan.

SERVES 4

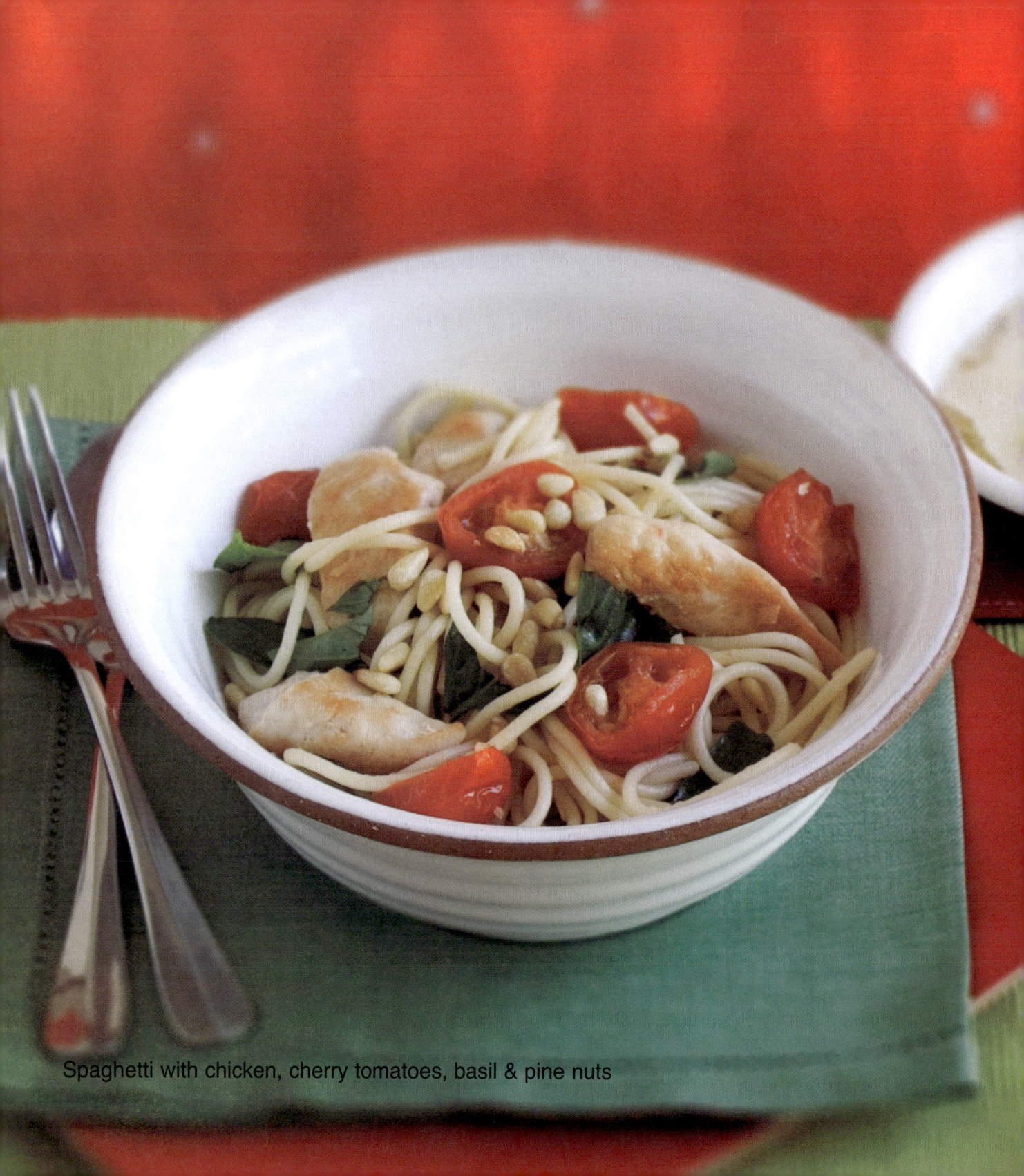

Spaghetti with chicken, cherry tomatoes, basil & pine nuts

Fat and essential fatty acids

While many of us shudder at the mention of the word, fat is a really important nutrient vital for health. Our body needs fat not only for stored and immediate energy, but also as insulation against heat and cold, protection of organs, supply of vitamins A and D, creation of hormones, and the maintenance of skin (dry skin is fat-deprived skin) and a healthy nervous and immune system. As with most things, it's about quality over quantity. All fats are not created equal. There is a group of fats called essential fatty acids, these are 'good fats' and are vital for health. Essential fatty acids may help in the prevention of certain cancers, diabetes, arthritis, autoimmune conditions, premenstrual syndrome and a host of other conditions. Essential fatty acids are found in fish, seeds, nuts, avocados, lean meat (especially wild game) and olive oil. Increase these foods while decreasing the foods containing the 'bad fats'—these include: pastries, margarine, most cooking oils, deep-fried foods, high-fat dairy and meat.

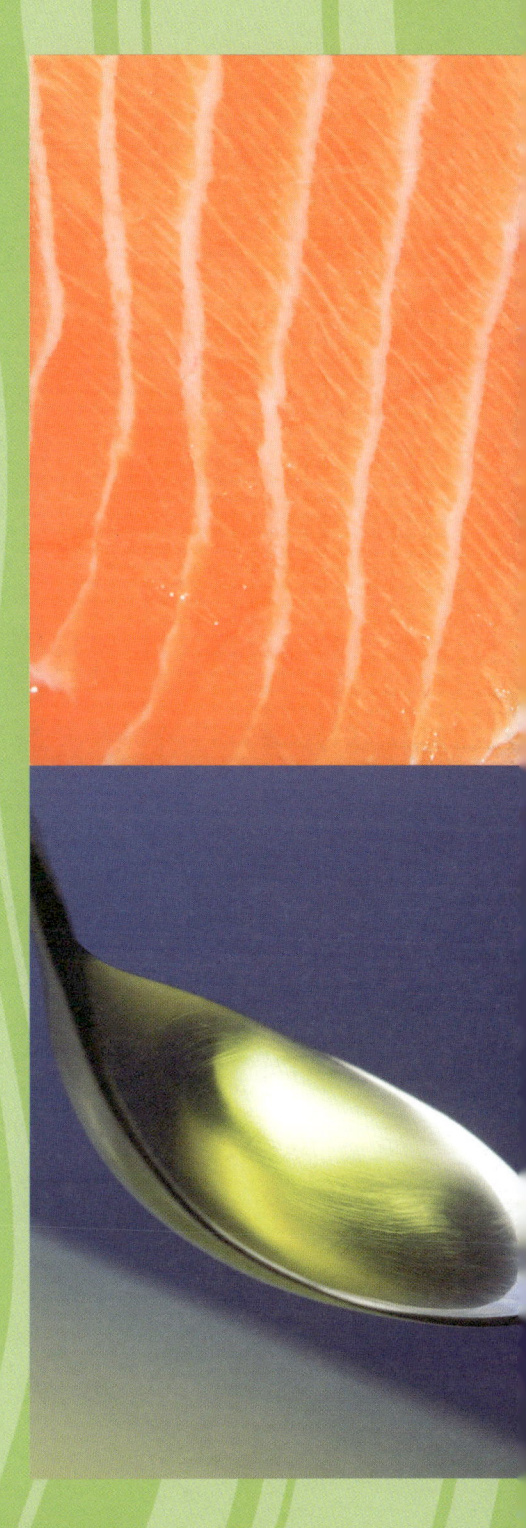

LAMB CUTLETS WITH MASHED POTATO, GARLIC GREEN BEANS & ROAST TOMATOES

I guess this is really 'meat and three veg', but it tastes and looks a lot better than that.

5 medium potatoes, peeled and cut in half
½ cup milk
sea salt and pepper
12 lamb cutlets, fat removed
1 tablespoon dried mixed herbs
500g/1lb 1½ oz green beans, topped and tailed
1 tablespoon olive oil
2 garlic cloves, crushed
8 roast tomato halves (p113)

Cook potatoes in rapidly boiling salted water until very soft (about 15 minutes). Mash, stir in milk and season to taste.

Rub lamb cutlets with a little salt and pepper and sprinkle mixed herbs on each side. Cook under a hot grill for 3 minutes on each side.

Steam beans until tender and toss with oil and garlic.

Serve cutlets with mashed potato, garlic beans and roast tomatoes.

SERVES 4

ROAST BEEF WITH MUSTARD, CHIVES & GARLIC

Rare roast beef should not be kept in the fridge for any longer than a day—as it is partially cooked meat, it could contain bacteria. Well-done beef can be kept for up to 3 days.

175g/6¼ oz jar wholegrain French mustard
½ cup finely chopped chives
2 garlic cloves, crushed
1kg/2lb 3¼ oz fillet of beef
sea salt and pepper

Preheat oven to 200°C/400°F.

Mix mustard, chives and garlic to a paste.

Rub beef with salt and pepper, then spread the mustard paste over it, making sure all sides are covered, including the ends.

Place in the oven and roast for 30 minutes (15 minutes per 500g) for medium-rare. If you like it well done, cook for another 15 minutes.

Remove beef from the oven, cover and keep warm for 5–10 minutes before slicing.

Serve with boiled baby potatoes and a green salad.

SERVES 4

ALMOST SHEPHERD'S PIE

Adding different vegetables to the meat component of a meal is a perfect way to increase kids' vegetable intake.

500g/1lb 1½ oz lean beef mince
1 onion, diced
2 celery sticks, diced
1 carrot, diced
1 cup frozen peas
1 cup broccoli florets
2 garlic cloves, crushed
1 tablespoon tomato paste
1 tablespoon soy sauce
1 cup hot water
1 bunch spinach, leaves only, chopped
sea salt and pepper

TOPPING
500g/1lb 1½ oz sweet potato
1 tablespoon of olive oil
sea salt and pepper
½ cup grated Parmesan

Preheat oven to 180°C/350°F.

Peel sweet potato and cut into 2cm/¾ in slices. Cook in salted boiling water for about 20 minutes or until soft. Drain off water and add 1 tablespoon of olive oil and mash. Set aside.

Heat a stir-fry pan on medium-high, add mince, onion, celery and carrot. Stir-fry until meat changes colour and onion is transparent (about 5 minutes).

Add peas, broccoli, garlic and tomato paste and stir-fry until the meat and vegetable mixture becomes quite dry (about 5 minutes). Add soy sauce and mix well.

Add hot water and cook for another 5 minutes.

Stir through spinach and season to taste.

Transfer to an ovenproof dish or 4 individual dishes.

Spread mashed sweet potato over the meat and vegetable mixture, dust with salt and pepper and score with a fork. Sprinkle Parmesan over the top.

Bake in oven for 30–35 minutes or until golden brown on top.

SERVES 4

CHILLI CON CARNE WITH AVOCADO & YOGHURT TOPPING

You could try this chilli con carne with either oven-baked corn chips on the side or on a bed of rice. This version has a large bean-to-meat ratio, which is a lot healthier than the usual recipe and a good way to get meat-lovers to eat beans.

1 onion, finely diced
300g/10½ oz lean beef mince
4 garlic cloves, crushed
3 teaspoons ground cumin
2 teaspoons chilli powder
1 tablespoon tomato paste
400g/14¼ oz can diced Italian tomatoes
2 x 400g/14¼ oz cans red kidney beans, drained and rinsed
1 cup hot water
sea salt and pepper

AVOCADO & YOGHURT TOPPING
2 ripe avocados
2 tablespoons lemon juice
sea salt and pepper
2 tablespoons natural yoghurt

2 tablespoons fresh, finely chopped coriander

Heat a heavy-based saucepan over medium heat. Add onion, beef and garlic, and cook for 10 minutes, stirring frequently.

Add cumin, chilli powder, tomato paste and tomatoes, stir and cook for 2 minutes.

Add kidney beans and hot water, stir and bring to the boil. Reduce heat to low, season to taste, cover, and simmer gently for 30 minutes.

To make the topping, mash avocados with lemon juice, salt and pepper. Stir through yoghurt and season to taste.

Serve chilli con carne with a dollop of avocado and yoghurt topping and a sprinkle of coriander.

SERVES 4

PENNE WITH TUNA, OLIVES & CAPERS

The leftovers from this dish are excellent in lunchboxes. I don't recommend cheese with this pasta.

400g/14¼ oz (or 4 cups) penne
1 tablespoon olive oil
1 onion, finely diced
2 x 400g/14¼ oz cans diced Italian tomatoes
1 cup pimento-stuffed green olives, cut in half
1 tablespoon capers, rinsed (optional)
2 x 425g/15oz cans tuna, drained well
1 teaspoon Tabasco
2 tablespoons lemon juice
2 cups finely chopped flat-leaf parsley
sea salt and pepper

Cook penne in rapidly boiling salted water until *al dente*. Drain well and set aside.

While pasta is cooking, heat oil in a stir-fry pan over a high heat, add onion and cook for 2 minutes or until softened.

Add tomatoes, olives and capers, if using, and cook for 2 minutes. Add tuna, Tabasco and lemon juice and cook for 5 minutes, stirring frequently.

Add penne and stir in a gently folding motion, making sure the penne is well coated with the sauce.

Add parsley and season to taste.

SERVES 4

BRAISED BEEF WITH MUSHROOMS, RED WINE & HERBS

Don't add all the liquids at once to braised meat dishes—that way, the meat gets a chance to cook in its own juice and the flavours diffuse much better.

1 tablespoon olive oil
1 onion, finely diced
500g/1lb 1½ oz lean diced beef, all visible fat removed
400g/14¼ oz can diced Italian tomatoes
2 garlic cloves, crushed
200g/7¼ oz button mushrooms, cut in half
2 tablespoons chopped thyme leaves
1 cup red wine
sea salt and pepper

Heat a heavy-based saucepan over medium heat, add oil and onion and cook until onion is transparent (about 3 minutes).

Add beef and seal on all sides. Add tomatoes and garlic, reduce heat to low and simmer gently for 20 minutes.

Add mushrooms, thyme and red wine, stir and simmer, covered, for 20 minutes. Season to taste.

Check after 20 minutes—if beef looks too dry, add a little (no more than ½ cup) hot water, stir and simmer for another 10 minutes. If there is too much liquid in the pan, increase heat and reduce the liquid to about ½ cup.

Serve with mashed potato or sweet potato and a green salad.

SERVES 4

Braised beef with mushrooms, red wine and herbs

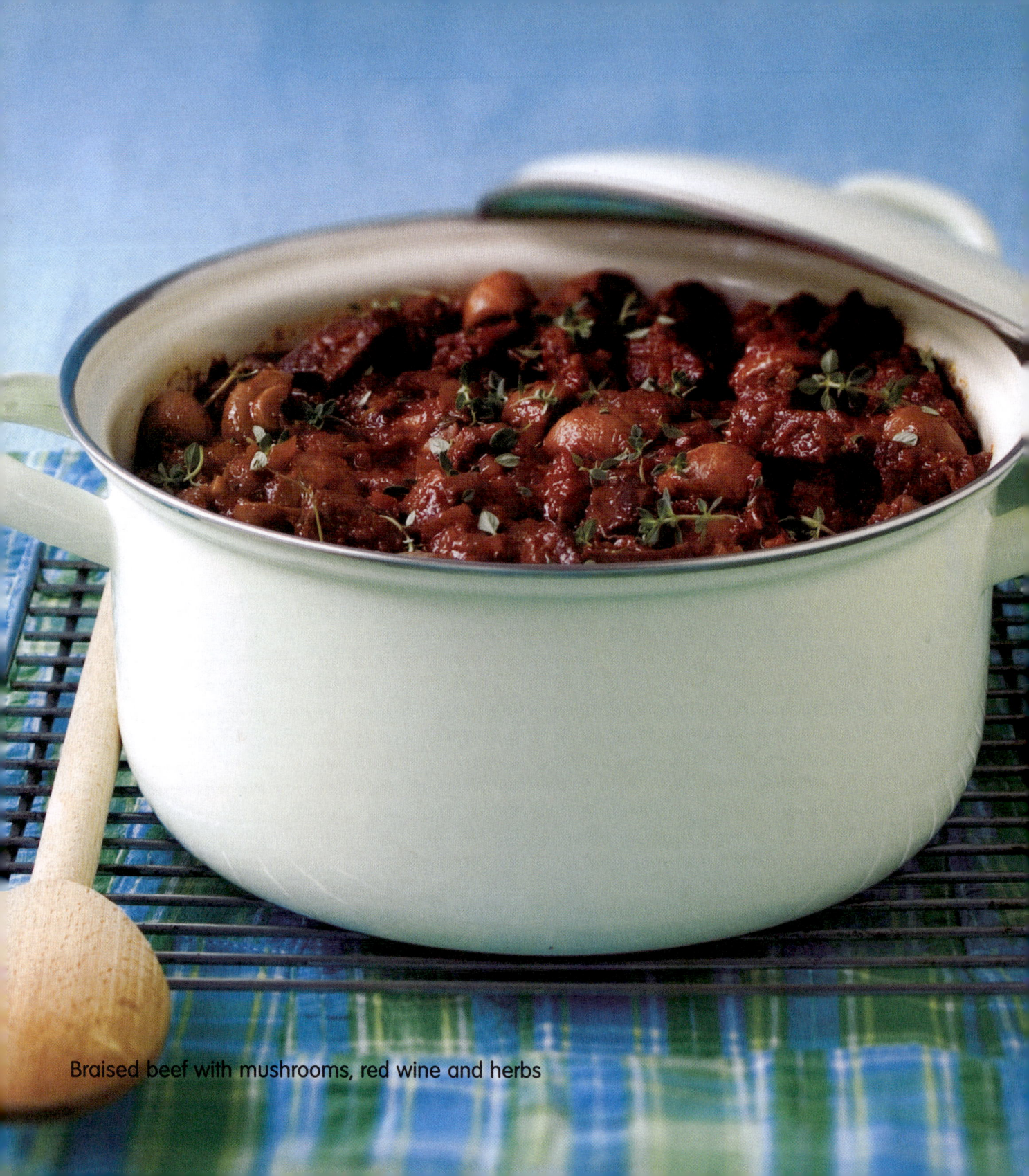

Broccoli

Along with cabbage, cauliflower, turnips and other members of the Cruciferous family, broccoli contains cancer-preventing components called indoles (which are believed to offer protection against breast cancer, in particular, because of their effect on oestrogen metabolism). Available year-round, broccoli brims with beta-carotene, a known inhibitor of cancer cells. An excellent source of iron, vitamin C and folate, it also benefits sufferers of chronic fatigue, anaemia and stress.

The Cruciferous vegetables are also high in soluble fibre, which is good for heart disease, constipation, diverticulitis and diabetes.

Broccoli can be juiced (diluted is best), eaten raw in a mixed salad, lightly steamed, stir-fried and used in soups. Its florets, stalks and leaves are all edible. But be warned: not only is broccoli unpalatable when overcooked, it's nutritional value plummets.

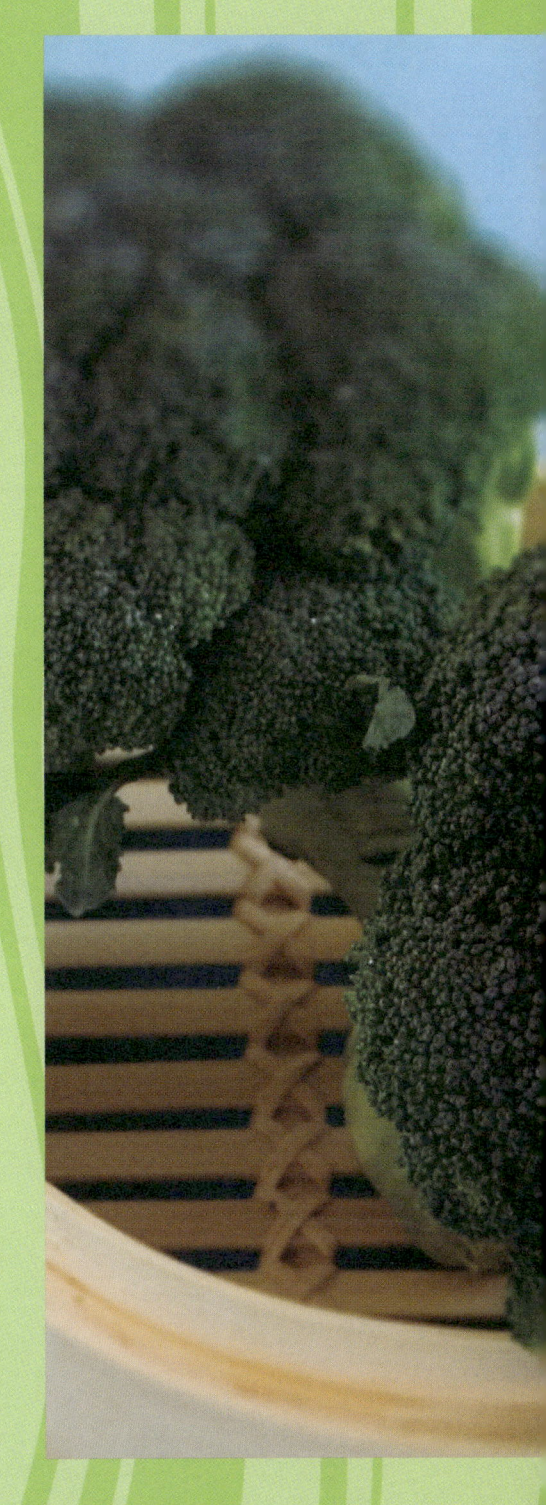

VEAL SHANKS

This is my version of osso bucco. The authentic version is a little too fiddly for me and it involves a fair bit of frying, which I try to avoid whenever possible.

4 veal shanks
1 onion, peeled and cut in half
2 bay leaves
1 cup tomato purée
½ cup red wine
1 tablespoon olive oil
grated zest of 1 lemon
2 garlic cloves, finely diced
1 tablespoon chopped thyme leaves
sea salt and pepper
1 tablespoon finely chopped flat-leaf parsley

Preheat oven to 180°C/350°F.

Line a small roasting tin with foil (this is for easy cleaning later). Place veal shanks in the roasting tin and add onion and bay leaves.

In a bowl or jug, combine tomato purée, wine, oil, lemon zest, garlic, thyme and salt and pepper. Pour over the veal shanks.

Cover the tin tightly with another sheet of foil, to keep the meat from drying out.

Bake in the oven for about 1½ hours—the meat will be falling off the bone.

Serve with parsley on top and lots of mixed vegetables on the side.

SERVES 4

CHICKPEA CURRY

You can make your own curry paste if you like, but there are so many good-quality ready-made ones (with good ingredients) don't bother.

1 tablespoon olive oil
1 onion, finely diced
1 eggplant, diced
2 x 400g/14 1/4 oz cans chickpeas, drained and rinsed
400g/14 1/4 oz can diced Italian tomatoes
100g/3 1/2 oz okra, trimmed and cut up
150g/5 1/4 oz green beans, topped and tailed
1 x 500g/1lb 1 1/2 oz sweet potato, diced
4 tablespoons rogan josh curry paste
3 cups hot water
2 cups firm tofu, diced
1 cup finely chopped coriander
sea salt and pepper

Heat a large, heavy-based saucepan over medium heat, add oil, onion and eggplant, and cook for about 2 minutes or until the onion is translucent and the eggplant has absorbed the oil.

Add chickpeas, tomatoes, okra, green beans, sweet potato and curry paste. Cook for another 2 minutes, stirring frequently.

Add water and bring to the boil. Reduce heat and simmer gently for 20 minutes or until vegetables are cooked. They should be on the soft rather than the crisp side.

Stir through tofu and coriander and season to taste. Cook for another 5 minutes.

Serve on a bed of steamed basmati rice.

SERVES 4

Chickpea curry

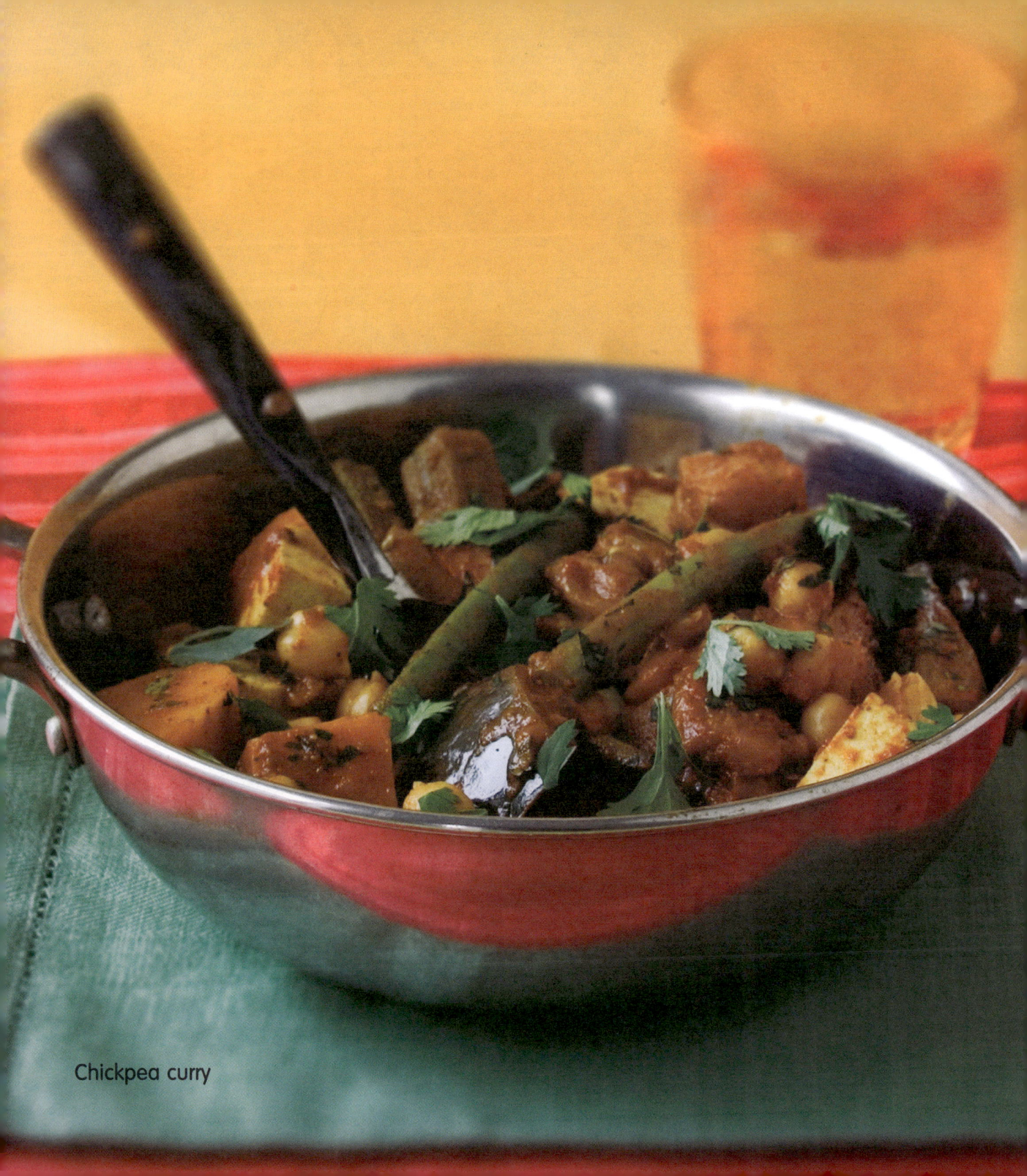

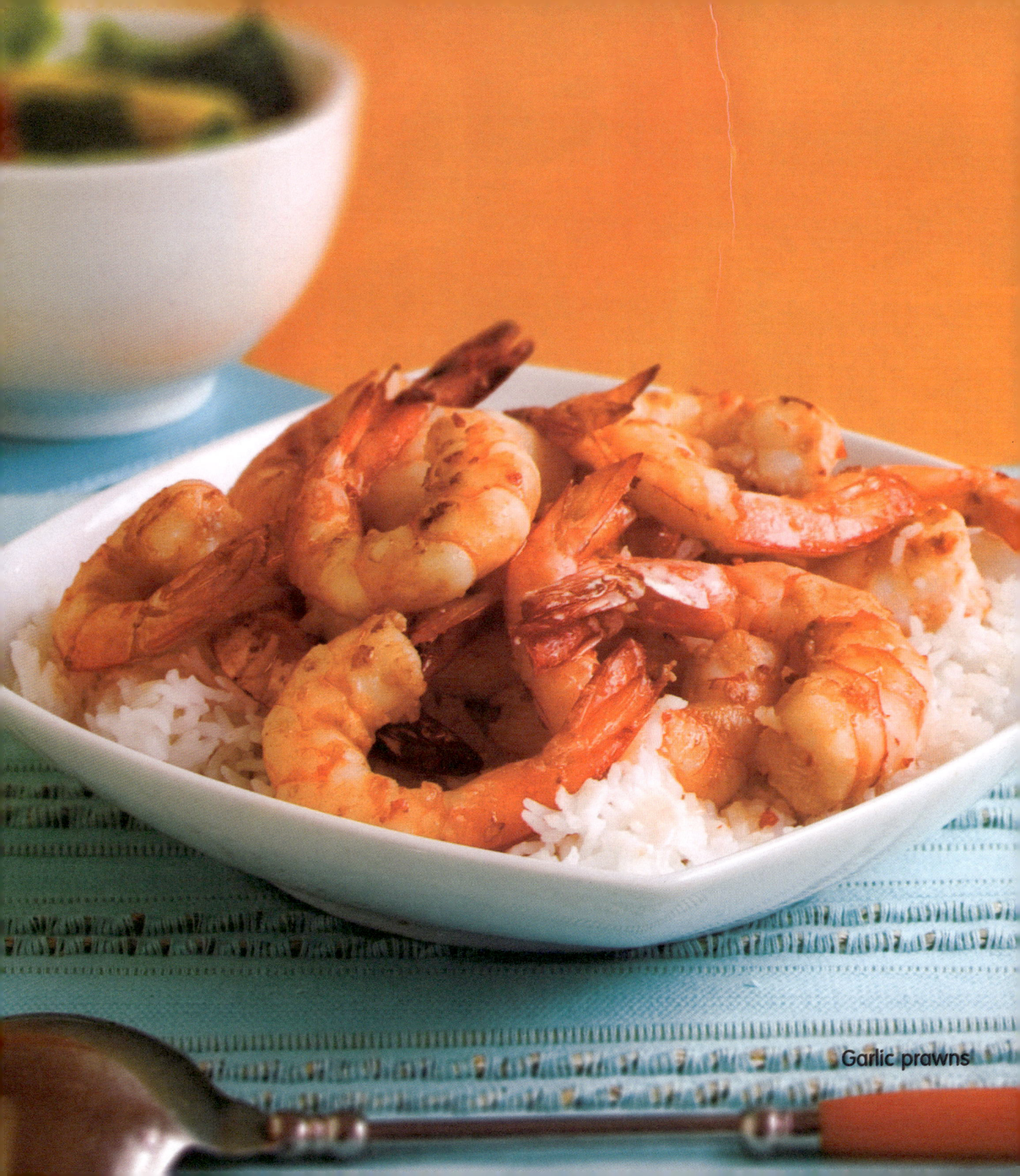

Garlic prawns

GARLIC PRAWNS

This is the Mediterranean version of garlic prawns. For the Asian version, add some Asian greens to the pan, a little splash of sesame oil and some cashews or peanuts.

32 medium green prawns, peeled and deveined
¼ cup olive oil
4 garlic cloves, crushed
1 teaspoon chilli paste
sea salt
1 lemon, quartered

Mix prawns with oil, garlic, chilli paste and salt.

Heat a large stir-fry pan on high, add prawns and stir-fry quickly until they turn red (about 2 minutes).

Serve on a bed of steamed rice with a lemon wedge on the side. A side salad of cos lettuce, fennel, onion, tomato and olives is delicious with this dish.

SERVES 4

GREAT NORTHERN BEANS WITH RICE

This was my father's favourite dish, so it was cooked often in our house. It's delicious hot or cold. My father's favourite version was the hot one with rice, whereas my mother and I preferred the cold version with a squeeze of lemon juice on top.

500g/1lb 1½ oz dried great northern beans
2 tablespoons olive oil
1 onion, finely diced
2 carrots, peeled and cut thinly into semicircles
2 garlic cloves, finely diced
1 teaspoon sugar
6 cups water
1 tablespoon tomato paste
sea salt and pepper
½ cup finely chopped flat-leaf parsley
rice, to serve

Place beans in a large bowl, cover with cold water and soak for a minimum of 6 hours or overnight.

Drain beans, place in a saucepan, cover with cold water and bring to the boil. Reduce heat to low and simmer for 5 minutes. Drain, rinse under cold running water and set aside to drain.

Heat oil in a large, heavy-based saucepan, add onion and cook for 5 minutes or until transparent but not brown.

Add beans, carrot, garlic, sugar and water and bring to the boil.

Stir in tomato paste, salt and pepper, reduce heat to low and simmer gently until beans are tender and most of the water is absorbed (about 45 minutes). The beans shouldn't be crunchy and the consistency should be about the same as baked beans.

Serve the beans on a bed of steamed rice with parsley on top.

SERVES 4

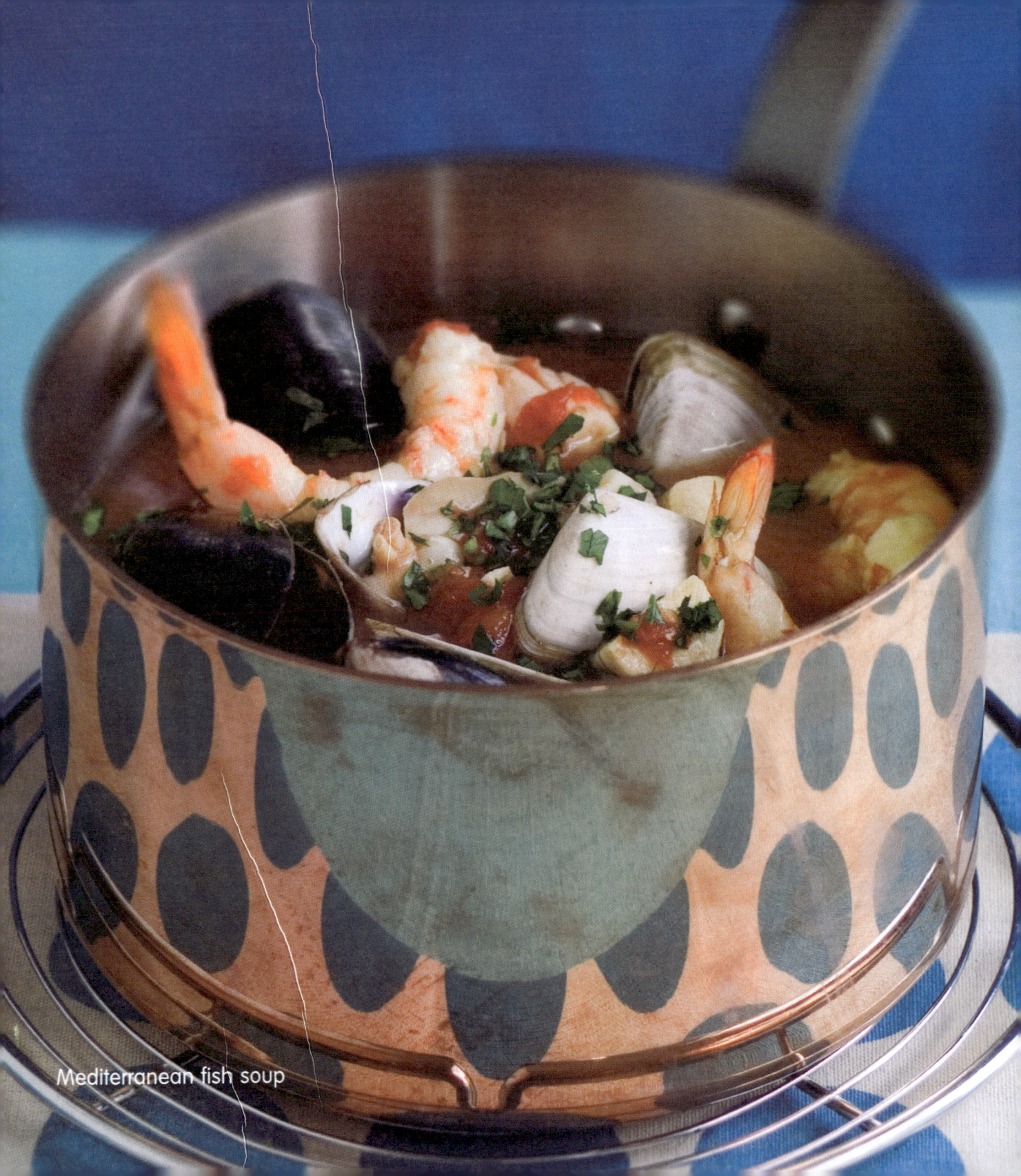

Mediterranean fish soup

MEDITERRANEAN FISH SOUP

Don't be put off by the two cooking stages. This is an extremely easy yet finger-licking good soup (more like a stew really). Make it on the weekend and serve it with a side salad in separate plates. You will need a bowl on the table for empty shells and some extra paper napkins. Young children may find the shellfish a bit difficult to manage, so you might have to help them.

FISH STOCK
½ cup olive oil
2 onions, chopped
3 garlic cloves, crushed
4 celery sticks with leaves, chopped
4 fish heads
8 sprigs each of thyme, oregano and parsley
3 bay leaves
8 whole black peppercorns
2 cups dry white wine
6 cups water

SOUP
2 x 400g/14¼ oz cans diced Italian tomatoes
1 tablespoon tomato paste
1 teaspoon powdered saffron
1kg/2lb 3¼ oz boneless, firm flesh fish fillets, cut into bite-sized pieces
20 green prawns, shelled and deveined
24 mussels, washed, scrubbed and debearded
24 pippies or clams, washed and scrubbed
sea salt and pepper
1 cup finely chopped flat-leaf parsley

Method on next page.

MEDITERRANEAN FISH SOUP (continued)

To make the fish stock, heat oil in a large, heavy-based saucepan over medium heat. Add onion, garlic and celery, and cook for about 5 minutes (don't brown).

Add fish heads, thyme, oregano, parsley, bay leaves, peppercorns, wine and water. Bring to the boil, reduce heat, cover and simmer gently for 45 minutes.

Strain fish stock through a fine sieve, and discard fish heads and vegetables.

Set aside to cool to room temperature, then cover and refrigerate.

To make the soup, pour stock into a large, heavy-based saucepan.

Add tomatoes, tomato paste and saffron and bring to the boil. Reduce heat, cover and simmer gently for 20 minutes.

Add fish and shellfish, cover and simmer until fish is cooked (about 5 minutes) or until fish is white and mussels have opened. Discard any mussels that haven't opened up.

Season to taste and transfer soup to a large serving bowl. Sprinkle with parsley and serve at the table.

SERVES 4

LENTIL STEW

I don't quite have '101 ways with lentils' but I'm getting there—I love them and they are so easy to prepare.

500g/1lb 1½ oz dried brown or green lentils
2 tablespoons olive oil
1 onion, finely diced
2 celery sticks, diced
1 large carrot, diced
2 small red chillies, deseeded and finely chopped
1 tablespoon chopped thyme leaves
1 capsicum, diced
1 large zucchini, diced
2 garlic cloves, crushed
400g/14¼ oz can diced Italian tomatoes
5 cups hot water
1 tablespoon tomato paste
sea salt and pepper
½ cup finely chopped flat-leaf parsley

Place lentils in a saucepan, cover with cold water and bring to the boil. Reduce heat to low and simmer for 5 minutes. Drain, rinse under cold running water and set aside to drain.

Heat oil in a large heavy-based saucepan, add onion, celery, carrot, chilli and thyme. Cook for a few minutes, stirring from time to time, until the onion is transparent

Add lentils, capsicum, zucchini, garlic and tomatoes and stir well. Add water and bring to the boil.

Stir in tomato paste, reduce heat to low and simmer gently until vegetables are soft and most of the liquid is absorbed. This will take about 20 minutes. Season to taste.

Serve in shallow pasta bowls and sprinkle parsley over the top.

SERVES 4

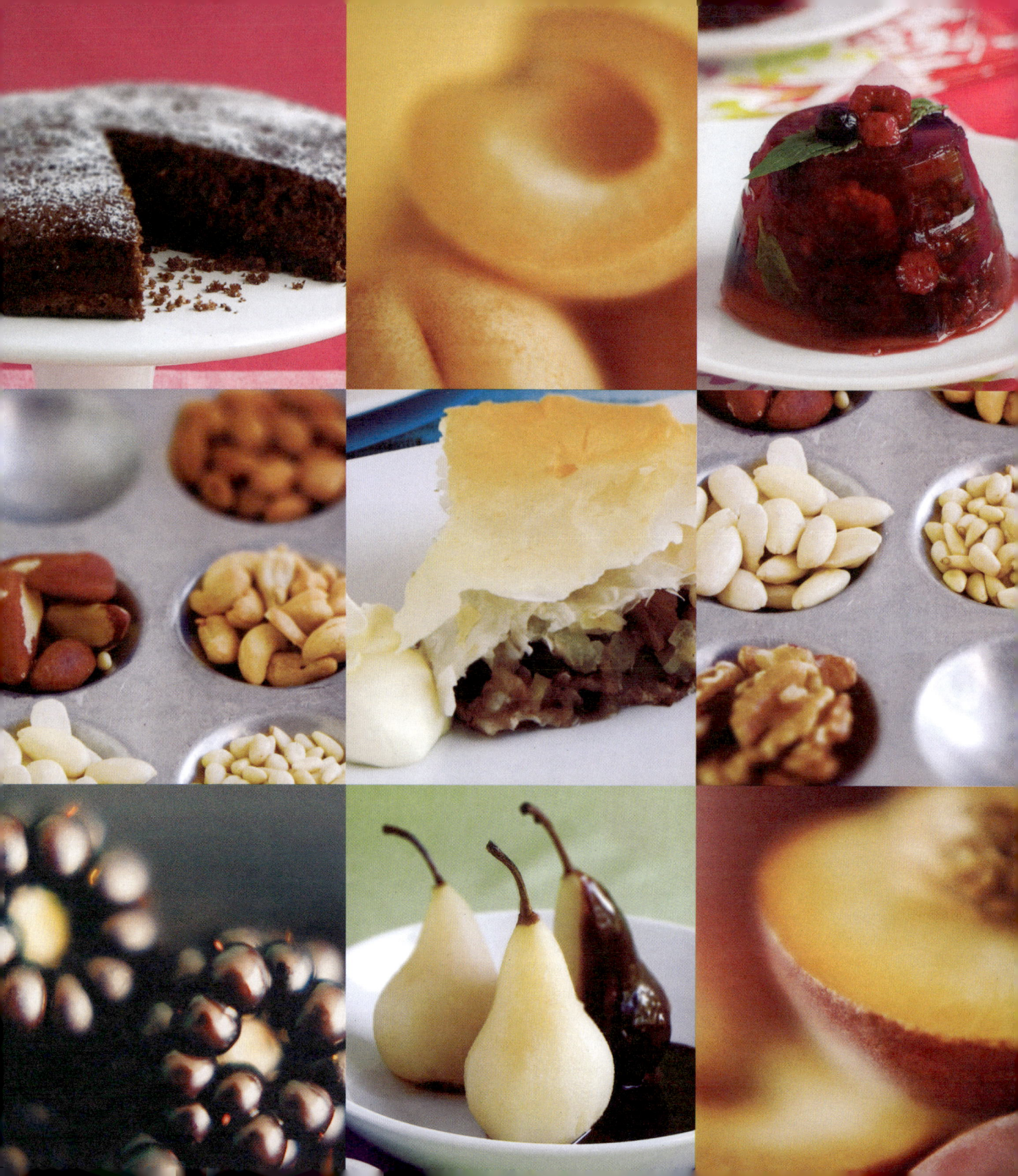

Treats

I have called this chapter 'Treats' because that's how desserts should be regarded. They are, as a rule, made up of empty calories which none of us needs. Having said that, it's nice to indulge now and again. I've made the following recipes as harmless as possible. Actually, some of them are even good for you but, even so, it's best to offer your family fresh fruit after dinner and keep 'naughty' desserts as a treat for the weekends.

APPLE & BLACKBERRY CRUMBLE

If by chance you have some crumble left over (this never happens in our house), you can keep it, covered, in the fridge for up to 3 days. This dish is also wonderful for breakfast.

400g/14¼ oz can pie apples (no-added-sugar variety)
150g/5¼ oz frozen blackberries
½ cup rolled oats
½ cup shredded coconut
½ cup brown sugar
½ cup melted butter
2 teaspoons ground cinnamon

Preheat oven to 200°C/400°F.

Combine apples and berries in an ovenproof dish.

Mix remaining ingredients in a bowl and spoon over the fruit. Press down firmly with the back of a spoon.

Sit the ovenproof dish on a baking tray, to catch the juices from the fruit if it bubbles over. Bake in oven for 25 minutes or until the top turns rich golden brown.

Serve hot or at room temperature with some yoghurt or ice cream.

SERVES 4

CHOCOLATE POLENTA CAKE WITH CHOC CHIPS

You just can't have a recipe book without chocolate recipes. As it happens, dark chocolate can be good for you, in moderation, of course.

6 eggs, separated
pinch of sea salt
½ cup honey
grated zest of 1 lemon
½ cup fine polenta, sifted
½ cup cocoa, sifted
½ cup dark choc chips
icing sugar for dusting

Preheat oven to 180°C/350°F.

Grease a 23cm non-stick springform cake tin.

Beat egg whites with salt until just stiff.

Combine honey, zest and egg yolks in a bowl and mix well.

Use a spoon to gently mix egg whites with egg yolk mixture.

Mix polenta and cocoa in a bowl, then fold into the egg mixture. Fold in choc chips.

Pour the batter into the cake tin. Place in the oven and bake for 40 minutes or until a skewer inserted in the middle of the cake comes out clean.

Set aside to cool in the tin.

Sift icing sugar on top of the cake when ready to serve.

SERVES 8

Chocolate polenta cake with choc chips

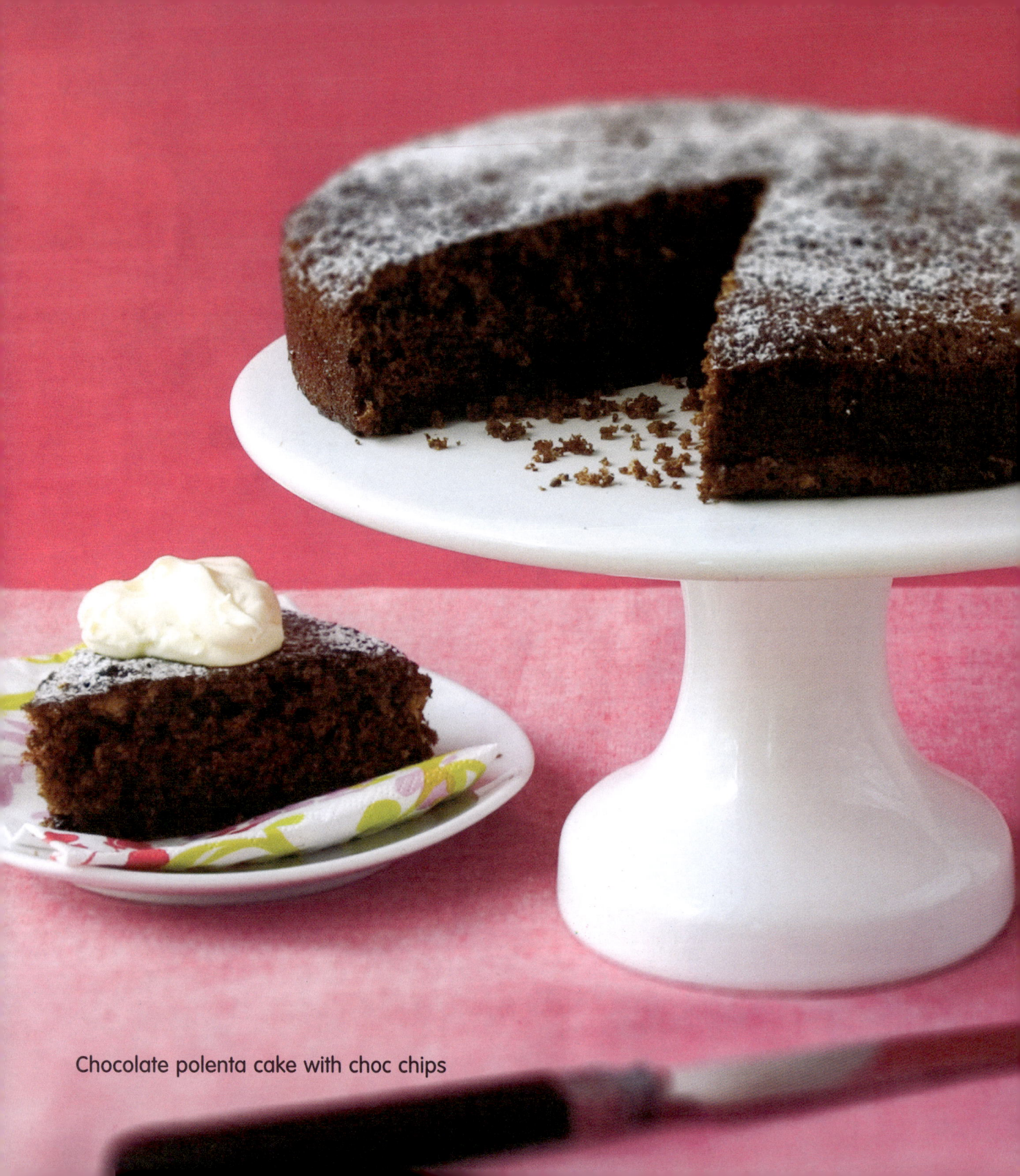

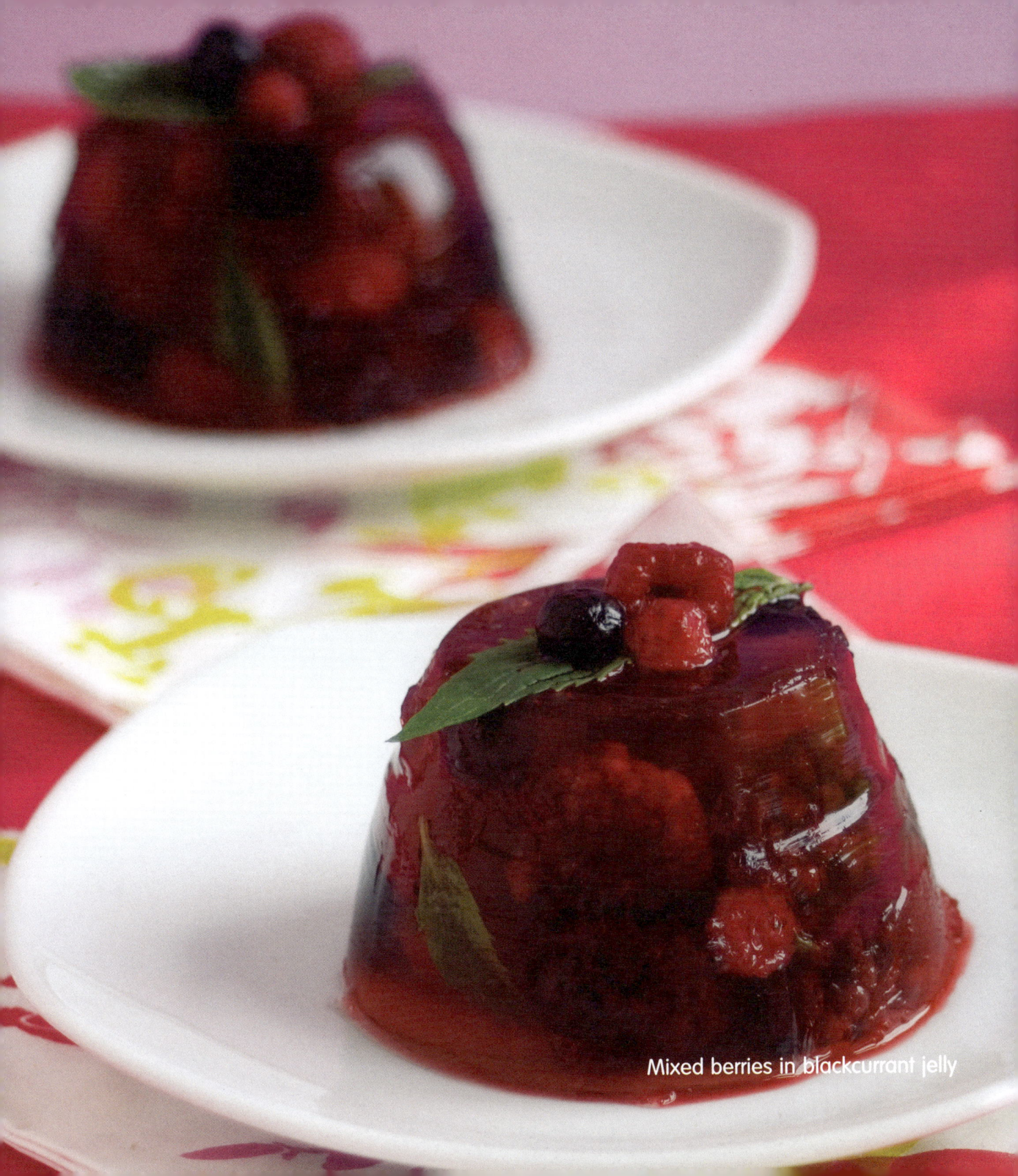

Mixed berries in blackcurrant jelly

MIXED BERRIES IN BLACKCURRANT JELLY

If you like a stronger blackcurrant flavour, use more fruit juice and less boiling water. You need ¼ cup of boiling water to dissolve the gelatine, but the rest can be fruit juice.

300g/10½ oz frozen mixed berries
20 tiny mint leaves (the little leaves on top of the stalks)
3 teaspoons gelatine
1 cup boiling water
1 cup blackcurrant juice
4 tablespoons double cream

Divide berries and mint leaves between 4 glass tumblers.

Dissolve gelatine in water. Add blackcurrant juice and mix well.

Pour the fruit juice mixture over the berries. Refrigerate until the jelly sets.

Serve berries in jelly with a tablespoon of cream on top.

SERVES 4

APPLE & WALNUT PIE

Filo pastry makes this pie very light, and strudel-like, but a lot easier to make.

1 cup canned pie apples, diced (no-added-sugar variety)
1 cup walnut pieces
2 tablespoons sultanas
1 teaspoon ground cinnamon
1 tablespoon melted butter
4 sheets filo pastry, cut in half (8 pieces in total)
1 tablespoon milk

Preheat oven to 170°C/335°F.

Mix apples, walnuts, sultanas and cinnamon in a bowl.

Brush a 23cm/9in pie dish with a little melted butter and line with 4 sheets of filo pastry, brushing the top sheet with a little more butter.

Spoon the apple and nut mixture onto the pastry base, spreading it evenly.

Cover the fruit and nut mixture with the remaining 4 sheets of pastry, brushing the first 3 pieces with a little melted butter. Brush the 4th piece of pastry (the piece that goes on the top) with a little milk.

Trim excess pastry around the rim of the pie plate. Brush the edges with milk so they adhere.

Place in the oven and bake for 40 minutes or until the pastry turns golden brown.

Serve warm or at room temperature. The pie is particularly good with vanilla ice cream, cream, or natural yoghurt mixed with a little honey.

SERVES 6

Apple & walnut pie

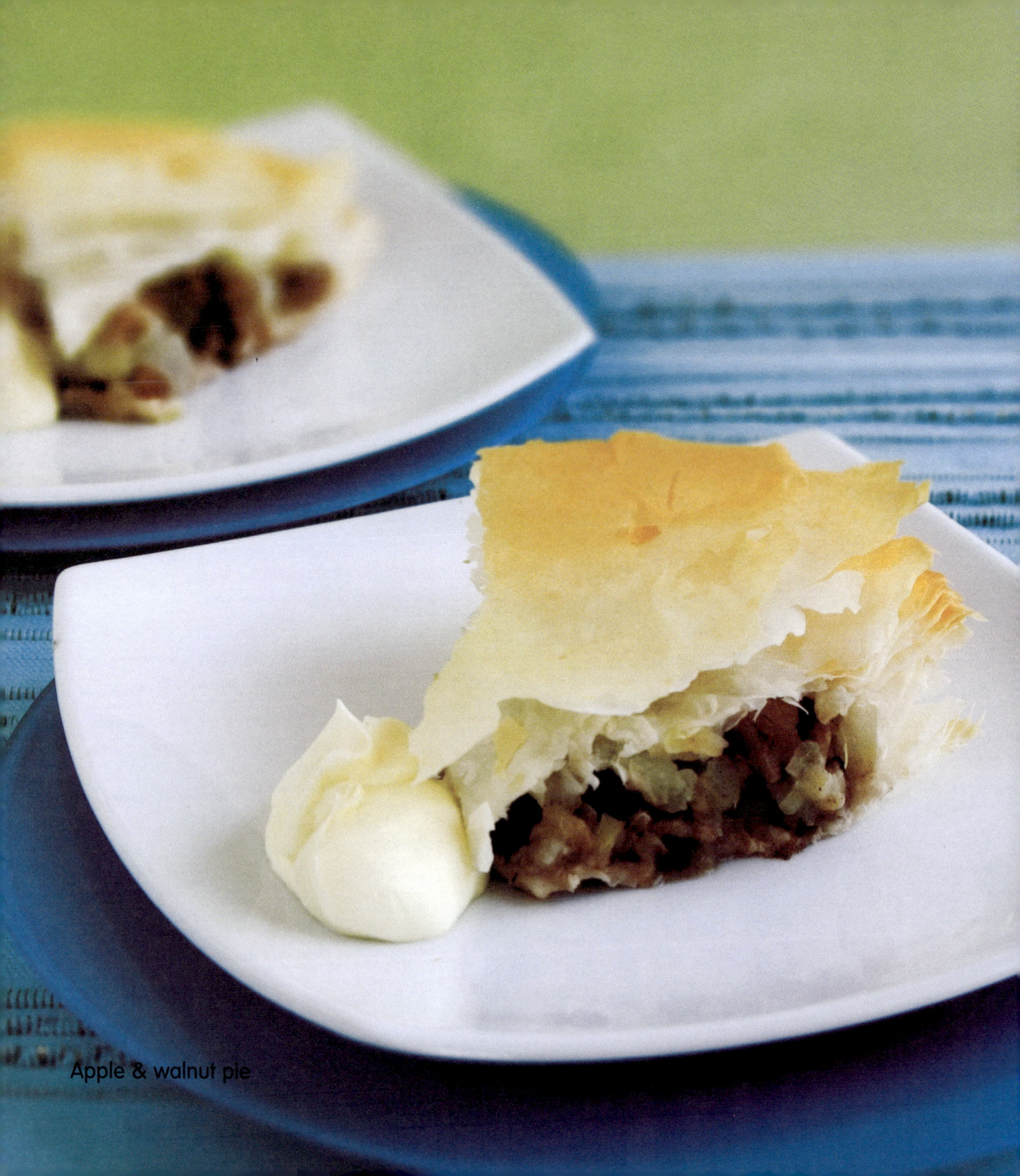

Nuts

One of the earliest foods humans consumed, nuts are bursting with nutrients. Yet it's only in recent times that nuts have been thoroughly researched for their health benefits. Studies reveal that nibbling on a mere 25g of nuts daily may reduce the risk of fatal heart disease by 45 per cent. Some researchers have even suggested that, because of their high unsaturated fat content, nuts are as effective as the statin drugs commonly used to lower cholesterol levels. Nuts also contain high amounts of protein, vitamin E, folate, fibre, calcium, potassium, magnesium and selenium.

All tree nuts are good for you, with each offering a different profile of micronutrients. Choose from almonds, Brazil nuts, hazelnuts, pecans, pine nuts, pistachios, walnuts, macadamias and cashews. Eat your nuts fresh, raw and unsalted. A fabulous breakfast is a mixture of your favourite nuts combined with sunflower seeds, linseeds, pepitas, sesame seeds, sultanas and currants. Mix them up and store in the fridge. For a great start to your day, just add some yoghurt.

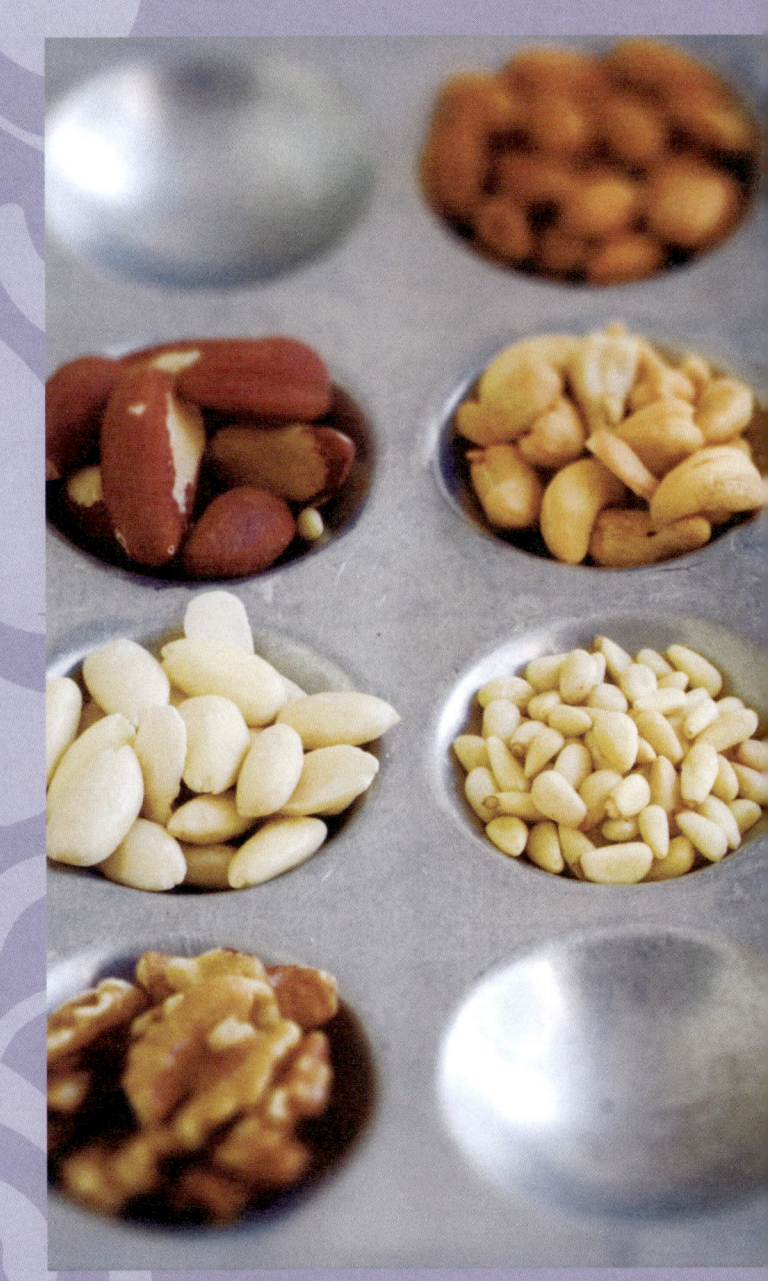

feelgood food 147

PUMPKIN PUDDING WITH NUTMEG & WALNUTS

When my mother cooks pumpkin, the pieces come out the same shape as when they went in and they are always cooked to perfection. When I cook it, they look a mess. So I decided to make some changes to the recipe to suit my capabilities. Any pumpkin is fine for this recipe.

1kg/2lb 3¼ oz pumpkin, peeled and cut into bite-sized pieces
¾ cup honey
¼ cup water
3 teaspoons gelatine dissolved in ¼ cup boiling water
1 teaspoon ground nutmeg
1 cup crushed walnuts

Place pumpkin, honey and water in a large, heavy-based saucepan, cover and slowly bring to the boil. Reduce heat to low and simmer gently for about 15–20 minutes until pumpkin becomes very soft and almost all the liquid has absorbed.

Set aside to cool.

Beat the pumpkin with an electric beater until smooth. Mix in gelatine and water.

Spoon mixture into 4 glass tumblers and chill in the fridge overnight.

Sprinkle over nutmeg and walnuts before serving.

SERVES 4

POACHED PEARS WITH CHOCOLATE SAUCE

As I'm sure you've heard many times before, when buying cooking chocolate, buy the best quality possible—the higher the cocoa component, the better the chocolate.

4 cups water
½ cup honey
4 pears, peeled, stems left on
2 cinnamon sticks
4 cloves
4 slices of lemon

CHOCOLATE SAUCE
100g/3½ oz dark cooking chocolate
100ml/3½ fl oz pouring cream

Place water and honey in a large, heavy-based saucepan on medium heat and stir until honey dissolves.

Add pears, cinnamon sticks, cloves and lemon slices. Bring to the boil, reduce heat to low and simmer until pears are cooked, about 20 minutes. Prod pears with a fork to check they're ready. They should be soft but not mushy.

Transfer pears to a deep bowl using a slotted spoon. Strain the cooking juices over the pears. Cool to room temperature, then refrigerate.

To make the chocolate sauce, break chocolate into small pieces and place in a bowl. Add cream and set the bowl over a saucepan of gently simmering water.

Heat chocolate and cream, stirring frequently, until chocolate melts and mixture looks shiny and creamy. Remove the bowl from the pan and set aside to cool.

Serve pears upright in 4 bowls, with a spoonful of chocolate sauce on the side.

SERVES 4

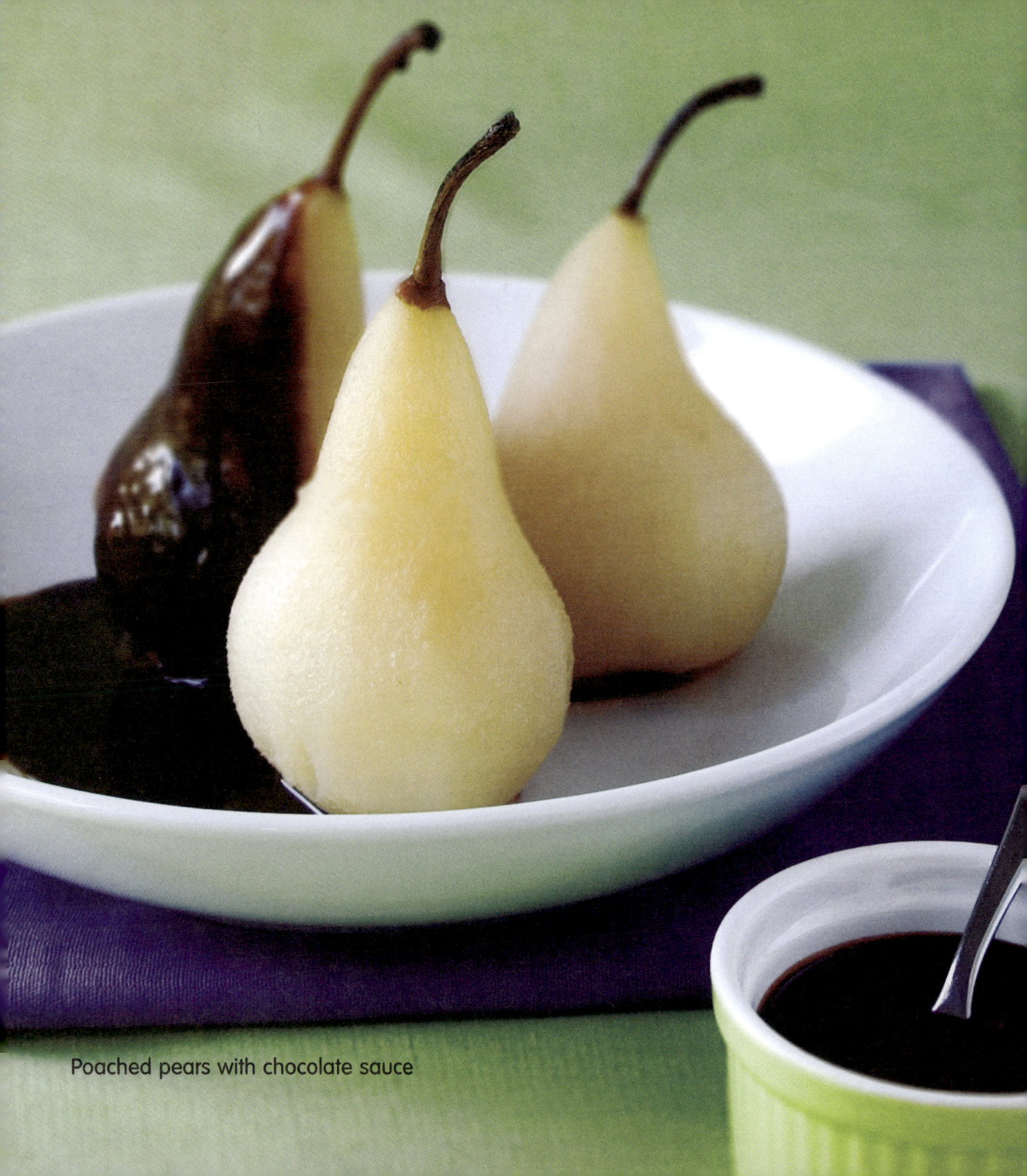

Poached pears with chocolate sauce

Cocoa

With the recent revelation that chocolate contains high levels of antioxidants, chocaholics around the globe breathed a sigh of relief. At last, their passion could be justified on health grounds—to a degree, at least. Antioxidants help prevent all sorts of conditions, including diabetes, heart disease, arthritis, cancer and even wrinkles. The antioxidants found in chocolate are called catechins, and the more cocoa in your chocolate, the more catechins. There are 53.5mg per 100g in dark chocolate, 15.9mg per 100g in milk chocolate, but none in white chocolate because it's cocoa-free. Apart from catechins, cocoa is also a rich source of minerals particularly iron and magnesium (420mg per 100g), which helps reduce muscle cramping, including menstrual cramps. Cocoa also contains iron, a mineral lost during menstruation and one that is needed for red blood cells to ferry oxygen around the body.

And there's more good news. Cocoa (not chocolate) can be useful in the treatment of high blood pressure because it acts as a mild diuretic and can dilate blood vessels. It can also benefit the sufferers of depression, thanks to the presence of phenylethylamine which is believed to trigger the release of feel-good chemicals.

But, unfortunately, the news isn't all good. In the case of chocolate (not cocoa), the beans are ground to a paste, sugar and fat are added. There are 520 calories contained in a 100g bar of chocolate, so when it comes to chocolate, moderation is definitely the key.

Note: drinking chocolate contains milk products whereas plain cocoa doesn't.

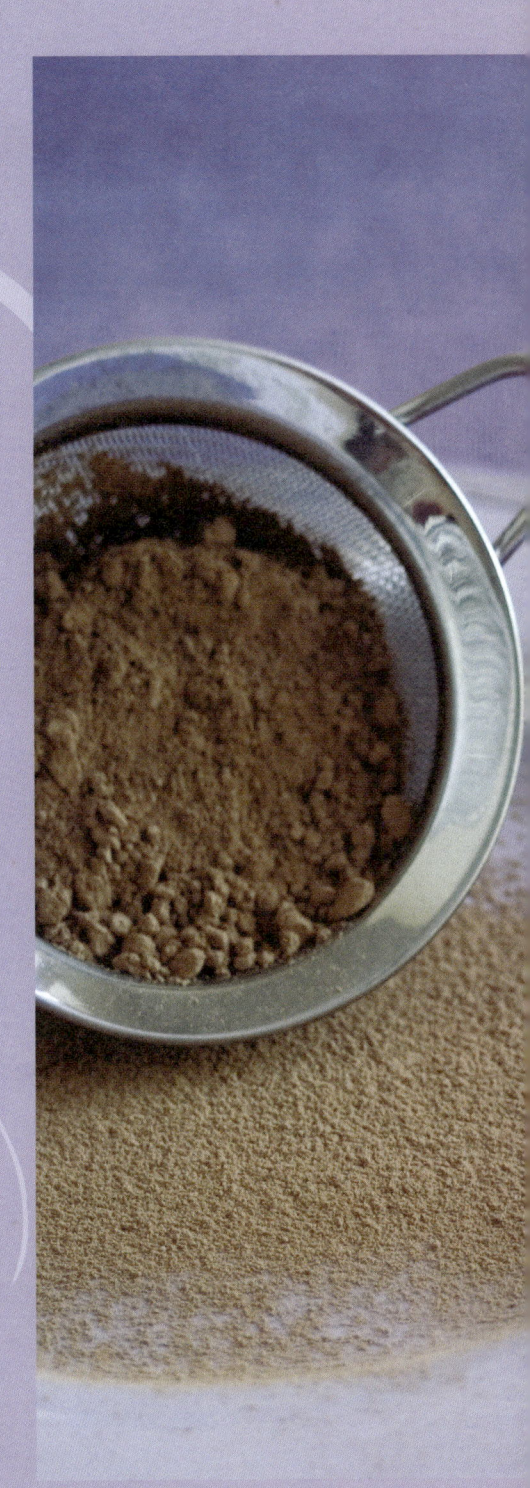

RICOTTA CHEESECAKE

This is as guilt-free as it gets when it comes to cheesecake.

1 cup cornflake crumbs
¼ cup LSA*
½ cup melted butter
1kg/2lb 3¼ oz fresh ricotta
1 cup honey
3 teaspoons gelatine dissolved in ¼ cup boiling water
¾ cup lemon juice
grated zest of 1 lemon

LSA, a mixture of ground linseeds, sunflower seeds and almonds, is available from health food stores and supermarkets. It's best stored in an airtight container.

Line the base of a 23cm/9 in springform cake tin with baking paper.

Mix together cornflake crumbs, LSA and melted butter. Press the mixture firmly into the base of the cake tin.

Combine ricotta and honey in a mixing bowl and beat with an electric beater until smooth.

Mix in dissolved gelatine mixture, lemon juice and zest, then pour mixture over the crumb base. Chill in the refrigerator overnight.

Remove cheesecake from the cake tin, place on a serving platter and serve with fresh berries.

SERVES 8

APRICOT & TOFU PUDDING

Tofu makes this pudding high in protein so it can double as a good breakfast choice or a snack.

415g/14¼ oz can apricots in natural juice
300g/10½ oz silken tofu
2 tablespoons honey
4 teaspoons gelatine dissolved in ¼ cup boiling water
2 tablespoons slivered almonds, toasted

Place apricots and their juice, tofu and honey in a blender and whizz until smooth. Add gelatine and mix well.

Pour mixture into 6 individual ½ cup-capacity moulds and refrigerate until set. This should take about 3 hours.

Dip the moulds in warm water for a few seconds, then turn out onto individual serving plates. Sprinkle each pudding with toasted slivered almonds before serving.

SERVES 6

feelgood food

STEWED APRICOTS WITH HONEY YOGHURT & ALMONDS

These apricots are delicious on cereals or served on their own as a snack.

250g/8¾ oz dried apricots
2 cups cold water
1 teaspoon vanilla extract
1 cup natural yoghurt
1 tablespoon honey
½ cup flaked almonds, toasted

Place apricots, water and vanilla in a heavy-based saucepan and bring to the boil. Reduce heat and simmer until apricots plump up and become soft (15–20 minutes).

Remove from heat and set aside to cool.

Transfer apricots and juices to a deep bowl, cover and refrigerate. They will keep in the fridge for 5 days.

Mix yoghurt with honey until well blended.

Serve apricots in 4 bowls, topped with a tablespoon of honey yoghurt. Sprinkle with toasted almonds.

SERVES 4

BREAD PUDDING

This pudding is quite filling, so I suggest you serve it after a light meal. You can store leftovers, covered, in the fridge for 2 days.

1 loaf good-quality fruit bread
4 eggs
3 cups milk
2 tablespoons honey
2 teaspoons vanilla extract

Slice the bread and remove the crusts.

Place slices of bread, overlapping, in an ovenproof dish.

Beat eggs, milk, honey and vanilla extract with an electric beater until well combined. Pour over the bread and let it stand for about 20 minutes.

Preheat oven to 180°C/350°F.

Place in the oven and bake until bread is puffed and golden brown and the milky mixture set (about 30 minutes).

Serve warm or chilled with fresh berries.

SERVES 4

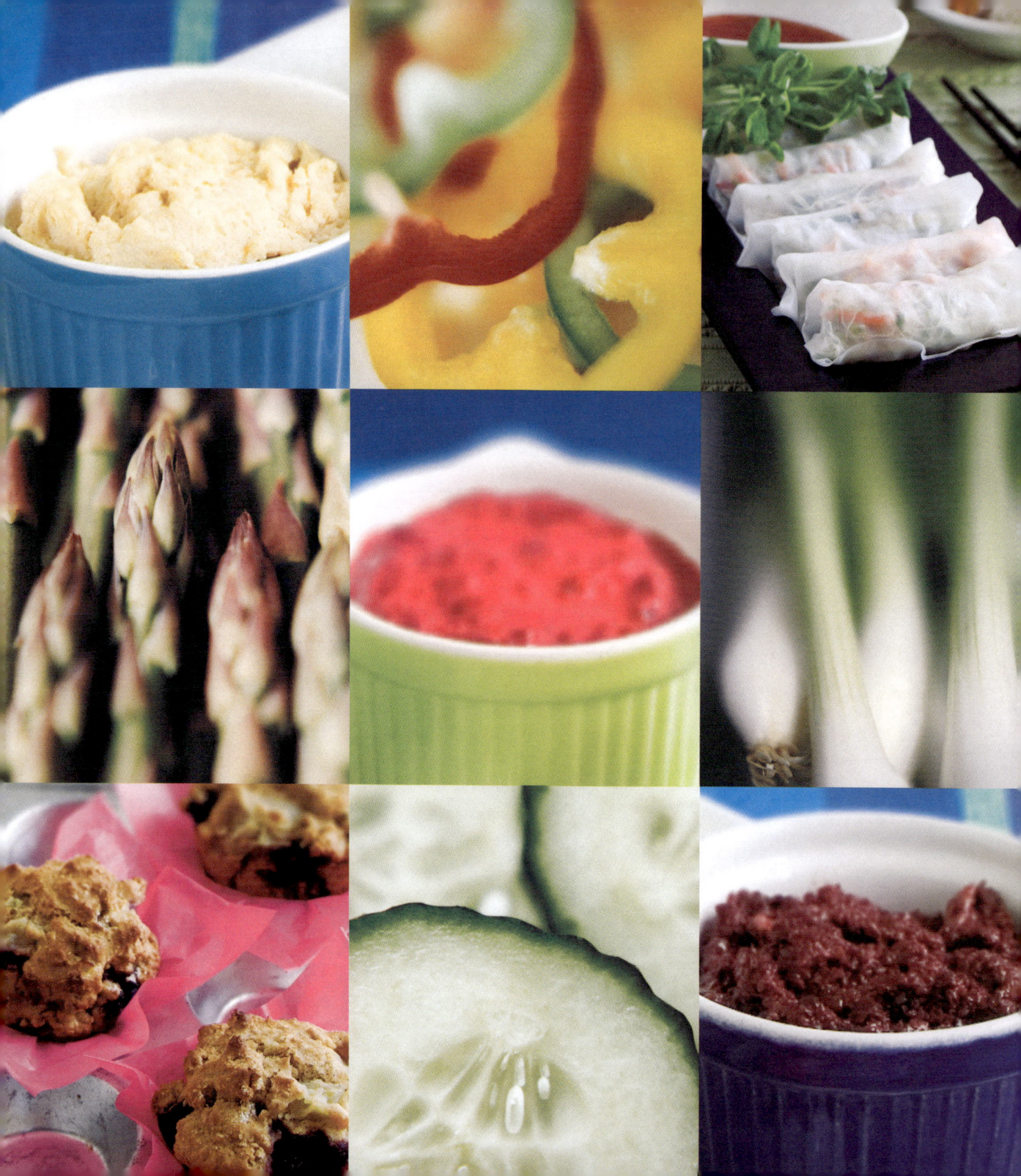

Snacks

I'm all for eating in between meals, just as long as you stay away from processed foods, sugar and saturated fats. You'll find plenty of healthy temptations on the following pages.

PUMPKIN & PEPITA MUFFINS

Buckwheat and brown rice have no gluten, making these muffins an ideal snack for anyone who's gluten intolerant. You can replace the buckwheat flour with wholemeal flour and the brown rice flour with white flour if you wish. You can also replace honey with molasses.

1½ cups buckwheat flour
1 cup brown rice flour
1 tablespoon baking powder
1 cup pepitas
1 cup cooked mashed pumpkin
2 tablespoons honey
1 tablespoon olive oil
1 cup milk
2 teaspoons vanilla extract

Preheat oven to 200°C/400°F.

Grease a 6 x ¾ cup-capacity muffin tin.

Combine buckwheat flour, brown rice flour, baking powder and pepitas in a mixing bowl.

Mix pumpkin, honey, oil, milk and vanilla in a separate bowl.

Pour the milk and pumpkin mixture into the flour mixture and fold in quickly with a wooden spoon. Don't overmix the batter.

Spoon batter into muffin holes. (An ice-cream scoop works best for this, giving an even distribution with the least amount of mess).

Bake in oven for 20–25 minutes. Insert a wooden skewer into the centre of a muffin to check it's cooked; if still wet in the middle, bake for a few minutes longer.

Turn out muffins onto a wire rack while hot. Leave to cool.

MAKES 6

EGGPLANT & TAHINI DIP

This dip is teriffic as a spread on sandwiches or accompaniment to grilled meats. Vegetable batons, toasted Turkish bread and breadsticks can all be served with this dip.

1 large eggplant, weighing about 500g/1lb 1½ oz
1 tablespoon olive oil
juice of ½ lemon
1 tablespoon tahini
¼ cup natural yoghurt
2 garlic cloves, crushed
½ teaspoon ground cumin
sea salt and pepper

Preheat oven to 200°C/400°F.

Prick the eggplant in about 6 places with a fork. Place in a baking dish and bake in the oven until the skin blisters, and the flesh collapses and feels soft (about 1 hour).

Remove eggplant from the oven, cut it open lengthways while still hot and allow the juices to flow out.

Scoop out the flesh and place in a bowl. Add oil, while the eggplant is hot, and mash with a potato masher. Add lemon juice and mix well.

Add tahini, yoghurt, garlic, cumin, and salt and pepper, and mix well. When completely cool, transfer the dip to an airtight container and store in the fridge for up to 5 days.

SERVES 4

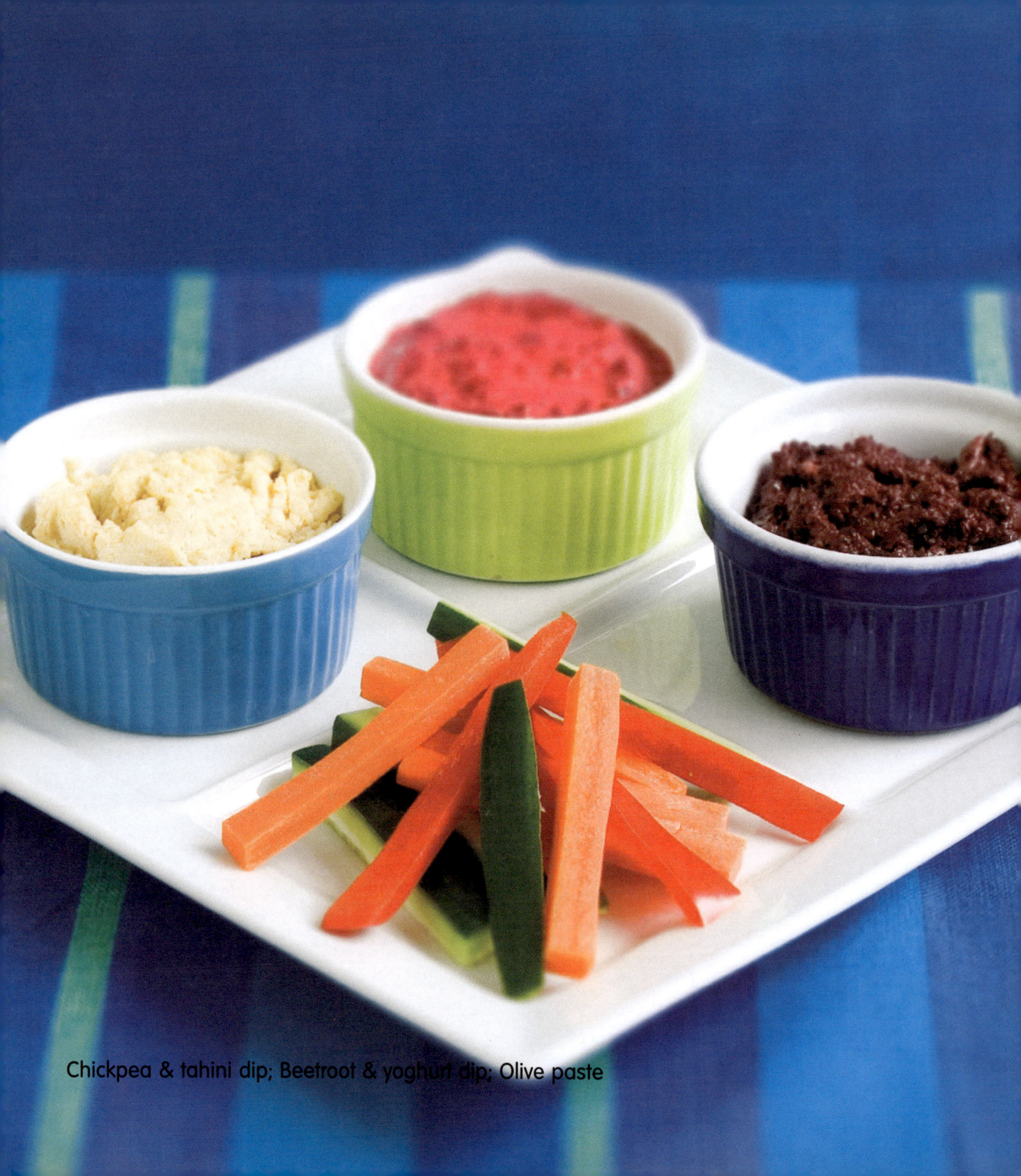

Chickpea & tahini dip; Beetroot & yoghurt dip; Olive paste

OLIVE PASTE

Olive paste makes a delicious spread for sandwiches, especially when combined with salad and cottage, cheddar or feta cheese. It is also a great dip for vegetable sticks or spread on crispbread.

375g/13¼ oz jar pitted kalamata olives, drained
1 tablespoon chopped thyme, oregano or rosemary leaves
1 garlic clove, crushed
juice of 1 lemon
½ red chilli, deseeded and finely chopped (optional)
freshly ground black pepper

Place ingredients in a food processor and whizz for 30 seconds.

Store in fridge in an airtight container for up to a week.

SERVES 4

CHICKPEA & TAHINI DIP

Good as a dip with pita bread or vegetable sticks, as a spread on sandwiches, as an accompaniment to grilled fish and meat, and as a salad dressing.

400g/14¼ oz can chickpeas, rinsed and drained
1 tablespoon tahini
1 tablespoon olive oil
juice of 1 lemon
2 garlic cloves, crushed
sea salt and pepper
¼ cup cold water

Place chickpeas, tahini, oil, lemon juice, garlic, salt and pepper in a food processor. Whizz for 15 seconds.

Scrape down the sides of the bowl and, with the motor running, start pouring water in a slow stream down the chute. Process until a smooth consistency is achieved. If too thick, add a little more cold water. Store in an airtight container in the fridge for up to one week.

SERVES 4

BEETROOT & YOGHURT DIP

This dip doubles as a delicious dressing for green salad. You might like to put it through the food processor to give it a smooth consistency. Try it with some Turkish or pita bread.

1 large beetroot, peeled and grated
1 tablespoon olive oil
1 tablespoon white wine vinegar
sea salt and pepper
½ cup natural yoghurt
1 garlic clove, crushed

Place beetroot in a bowl with oil, vinegar and salt and pepper. Mix well.

Mix yoghurt with garlic.

Combine dressed beetroot and yoghurt and garlic and mix well.

SERVES 4

feelgood food

OAT & SUNFLOWER-SEED COOKIES

These cookies are nutritious enough to eat for breakfast on those days when you've slept through the alarm clock.

1 cup rolled oats
½ cup shredded coconut
½ cup dried apricots, diced
½ cup sunflower seeds
¼ cup sesame seeds
2 eggs
¼ cup honey
1 tablespoon olive oil
2 teaspoons vanilla extract

Preheat oven to 160°C/325°F.

Line a baking tray with baking paper.

Combine oats, coconut, apricots, sunflower seeds and sesame seeds in a mixing bowl.

Whisk eggs, honey, oil and vanilla until honey dissolves.

Pour the egg and honey mixture into the bowl containing the dry ingredients and mix well.

Place dessertspoonfuls of the mixture onto the baking tray. Smooth each cookie with the back of a spoon.

Place in the oven and bake for 20–25 minutes, until cookies turn golden brown. Leave to cool on the baking tray for a few minutes, then transfer to a wire rack. Allow to cool completely. Store for up to a week in an airtight container in the pantry.

MAKES 16

RICE PAPER ROLLS

You can use any filling you wish in these rolls as long as you keep the ingredients reasonably dry. If the filling is too wet, the rolls will get soggy and be hard to handle.

8 rice paper sheets
1 cup salad sprouts (my favourite is broccoli sprouts)
1 carrot, grated
32 unsalted, roasted cashews
½ Lebanese cucumber, cut into sticks
½ red capsicum, cut into sticks
2 spring onions, cut into quarters lengthways
½ avocado, cut into 8 slices lengthways

Place a sheet of rice paper in a bowl of warm water for 10 seconds to soften. Transfer to a clean cutting board.

Pile a good pinch of salad sprouts in the middle of the rice paper and top with grated carrot. Then line 4 cashews on top.

Top the cashews with sticks of cucumber, capsicum and spring onion and a slice of avocado.

Fold one edge of the rice paper over the filling. Then fold the opposite edge over the filling, so that both ends of the roll are covered. Finish rolling the rice paper to enclose the contents. (This is easy as the damp and softened paper sticks without any problems).

Serve with a small bowl of soy sauce or sweet chilli sauce for dipping.

MAKES 8

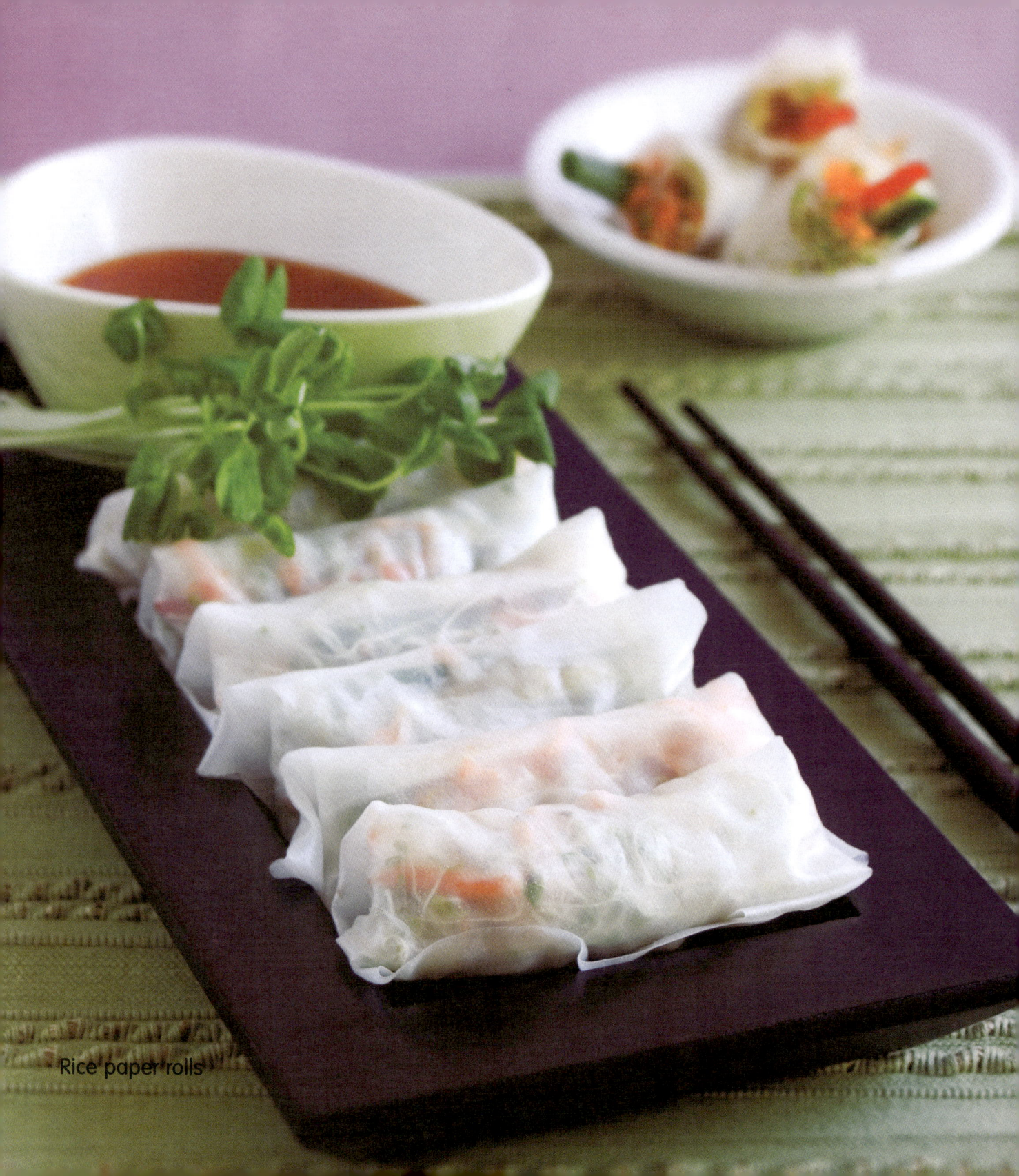

Rice paper rolls

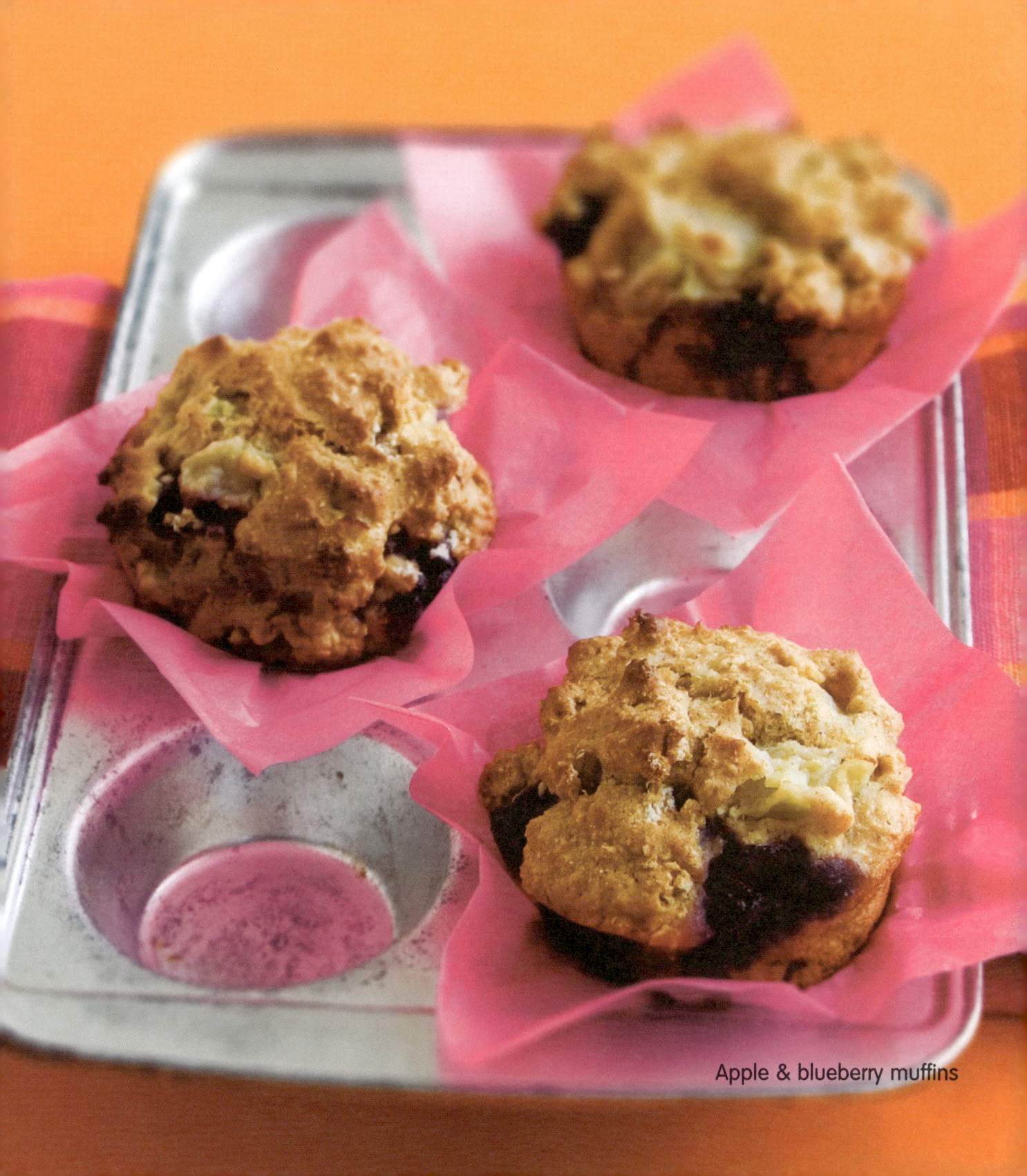

Apple & blueberry muffins

APPLE & BLUEBERRY MUFFINS

If you're after something healthy to tide you over until lunch or dinner, one of these delicious muffins will do the job.

2½ cups wholemeal flour
1 tablespoon baking powder
2 teaspoons ground cinnamon
1 cup canned pie apples, diced
1 cup frozen blueberries
2 tablespoons honey
1 tablespoon olive oil
2 teaspoons vanilla extract
1¼ cups milk

Preheat oven to 200°C/400°F.

Grease a 6 x ¾ cup-capacity muffin tin.

Combine flour, baking powder and cinnamon in a mixing bowl.

Mix apples, blueberries, honey, oil, vanilla and milk in another mixing bowl.

Pour the milk and fruit mixture into the flour mixture and fold in quickly with a wooden spoon. Don't overmix the batter.

Spoon batter into muffin holes using an ice-cream scoop.

Bake in oven for 20–25 minutes. Insert a wooden skewer into the centre of a muffin to check if it is cooked; if still wet in the middle, bake for a few minutes longer.

Turn out muffins onto a wire rack while hot. Leave to cool.

MAKES 6

CHOCOLATE & RASPBERRY MUFFINS

Store muffins in an airtight container in the fridge for up to 3 days. Warm them in the microwave for a minute, or in the oven for 10 minutes, before eating.

1 cup buckwheat flour
1 cup brown rice flour
½ cup cocoa, sifted
1 tablespoon baking powder
2 cups frozen raspberries
2 tablespoons honey
1 tablespoon olive oil
1½ cups milk
2 teaspoons vanilla extract

Preheat oven to 200°C/400°F.

Grease a 6 x ¾ cup-capacity muffin tin.

Combine buckwheat flour, brown rice flour, cocoa and baking powder in a mixing bowl.

Mix together raspberries, honey, oil, milk and vanilla in a separate bowl.

Pour the milk and raspberry mixture into the flour mixture and fold in quickly with a wooden spoon. Don't overmix the batter.

Spoon batter into the muffin holes using an ice-cream scoop.

Bake in oven for 20–25 minutes. Insert a wooden skewer into the centre of a muffin to check if it is cooked; if still wet in the middle, bake for a few minutes longer.

Turn out muffins onto a wire rack while hot. Leave to cool.

MAKES 6

SPICY AVOCADO MASH ON GARLIC TOAST

This is a fantastic quick snack when you're hungry. Served on bite-sized pieces of toast, it also makes a delicious nibbly for pre-dinner drinks.

1 large ripe avocado
2 teaspoons white wine vinegar
2 teaspoons lemon juice
few drops Tabasco
sea salt and pepper
1 garlic clove, peeled and cut in half
4 slices of sourdough bread, toasted

Scoop avocado flesh into a bowl and mash with a fork.

Add vinegar, lemon juice, Tabasco, and salt and pepper. Mix well.

Rub one side of each slice of toast with the cut side of the garlic clove.

Spread mashed avocado mixture on slices of toast.

SERVES 4

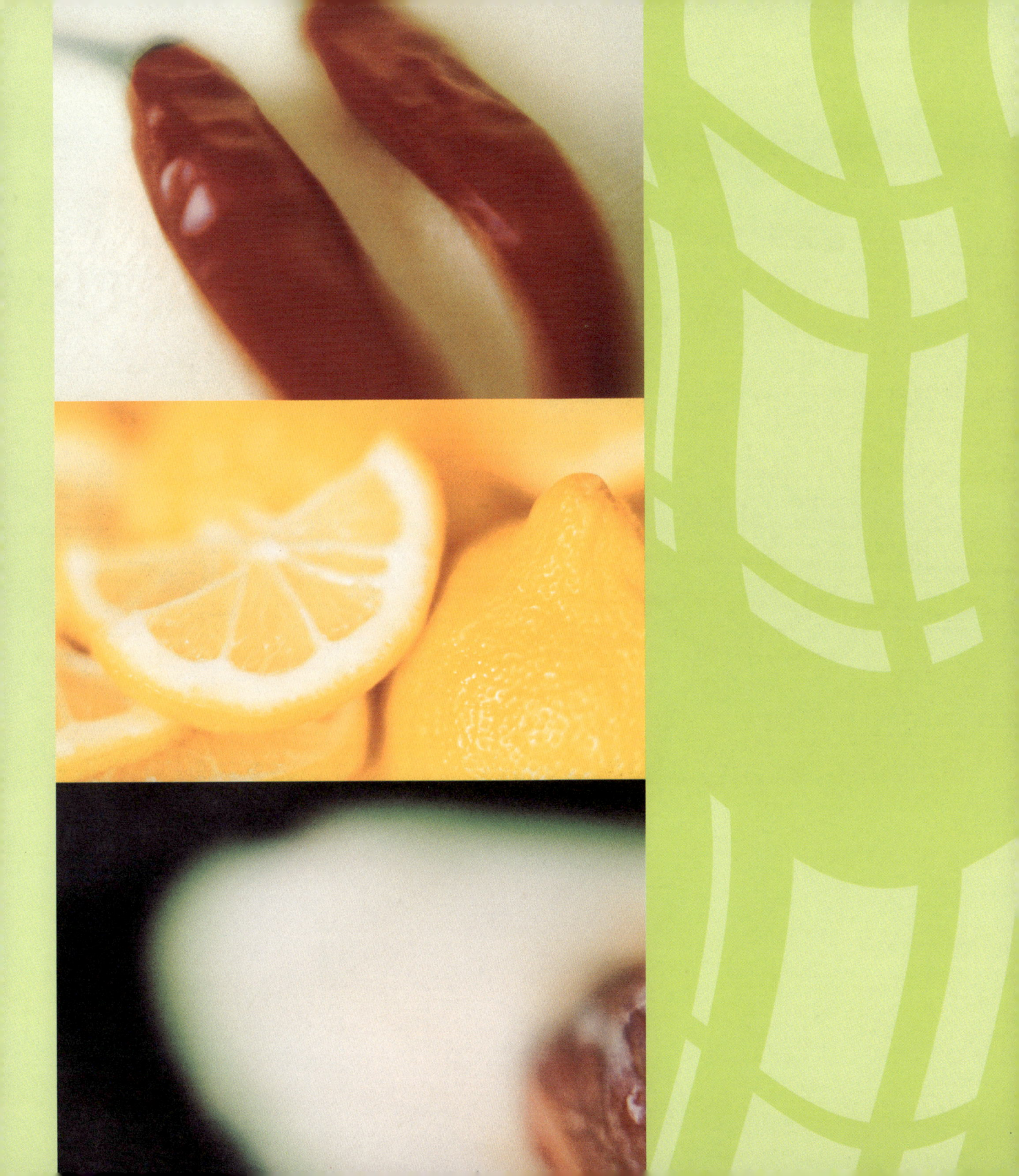

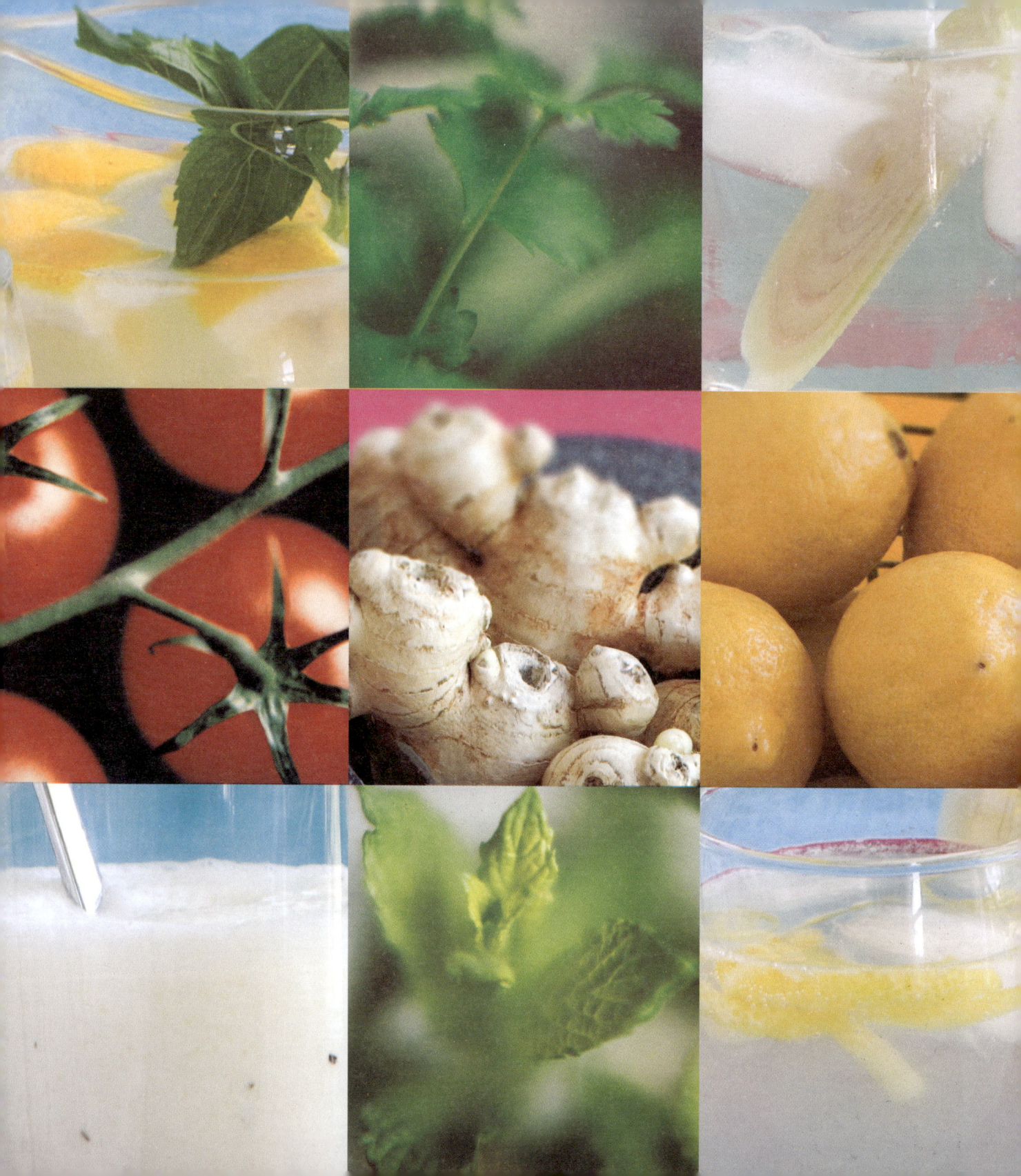

Drinks

Thirst is often confused with hunger. Of course, the best drink throughout the day is water, but why not extend your liquid intake to these healthy and refreshing drinks overleaf? But remember—if you are going to have a drink other than water, try not to have food with it. Try and avoid 'coffee and cake' or 'tea and biscuits'.

ICED SPICED GREEN TEA

This is a good alternative for those coffee drinkers who have been told to cut back.

1 tablespoon loose green tea or 6 tea bags
2 cinnamon sticks, broken in half
6 cloves
4 cups boiling water
1 tablespoon honey
4 slices of lemon

Place green tea or tea bags, cinnamon sticks and cloves in a teapot and top with boiling water. Set aside to infuse for 15 minutes.

Strain tea into a jug, stir in honey and lemon slices. Refrigerate for 2 hours or until chilled.

Place ice cubes in 4 glasses, add cold tea and a slice of lemon.

SERVES 4

HOT COCOA

Here's a drink for the chocolate lovers out there. Make sure you use cocoa powder, not drinking chocolate.

4 teaspoons cocoa powder
boiling water
hot milk, to taste
honey, to taste

Place a teaspoon of cocoa powder into 4 mugs.

Pour boiling water into the mugs, and stir well until cocoa dissolves.

Top with milk, add honey, to taste, and stir again.

LEMONADE WITH MINT LEAVES

My mother used to serve this on hot summer afternoons.

4 cups cold water
juice of 4 lemons
2 tablespoons honey
½ cup mint leaves

Pour water and lemon juice into a jug and stir well.

Add honey and stir until dissolved. If it tastes too sharp, add a little more cold water; if it needs to be sweeter, add a little more honey.

Add mint leaves and refrigerate for 2 hours or until thoroughly chilled.

Place ice cubes in 4 large glasses and top with lemonade.

SERVES 4

ICED LEMONGRASS TEA

The ultimate in refreshing drinks.

4 stalks lemongrass, very finely sliced
2 cups boiling water
2 tablespoons honey
2 cups soda water

Place lemongrass in a teapot, pour over boiling water, cover and set aside to infuse until cool.

Strain tea into a jug, add honey and stir well. Refrigerate for about 2 hours.

Place ice cubes in 4 glasses.

Stir soda water into the lemongrass tea and pour into the prepared glasses.

SERVES 4

Lemonade with mint leaves

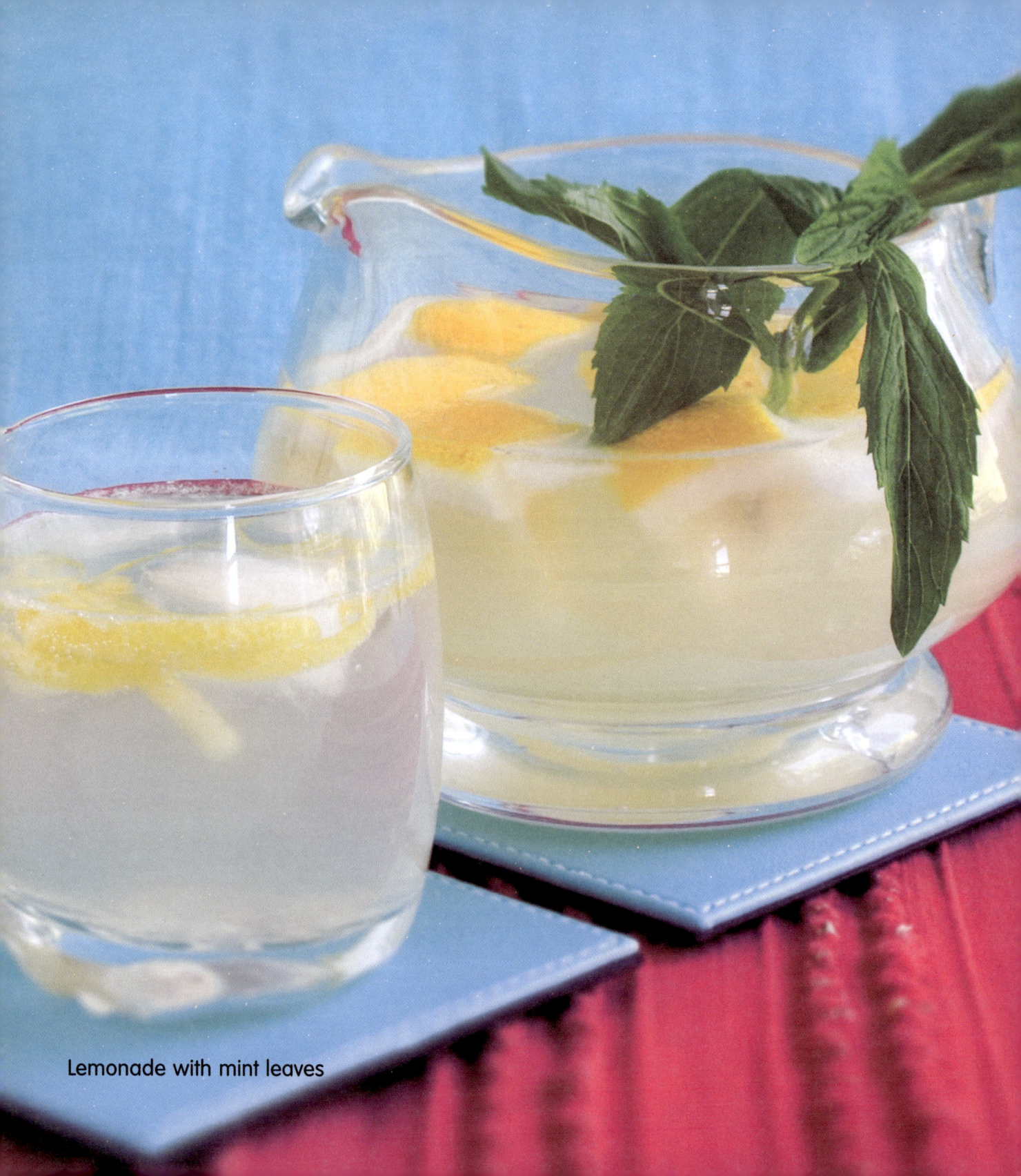

Lemons

Even before the formal identification of vitamin C, the humble lemon's efficacy in treating scurvy—the result of a diet lacking in ascorbic acid, another name for vitamin C—received wide coverage. It was so effective, in fact, that from the 18th century onwards, every English vessel that set sail for foreign lands had to, by law, carry lemons or limes.

Apart from brimming with vitamin C, lemons are rich in bioflavonoids (especially the peel and pith), potassium and magnesium.

When sipped in small amounts before a meal, lemon juice acts as an effective cleanser, stimulating the flow of bile from the liver. (Just make sure you rinse your mouth with water afterwards, as lemon juice can corrode tooth enamel.) Gargling diluted lemon is said to aid sore throats and gum disease. The fruit's antiseptic powers not only help ward off colds and flu.

Lemons are also effective antioxidants—squeeze a little over other fruit and vegetables to prevent browning and act as a preservative. Because vitamin C increases iron absorption, add lemon to green vegetables, soups and meat dishes. Those prone to queasiness, gallstones, constipation, or digestive or skin problems, should boost the amount of lemon in their diet.

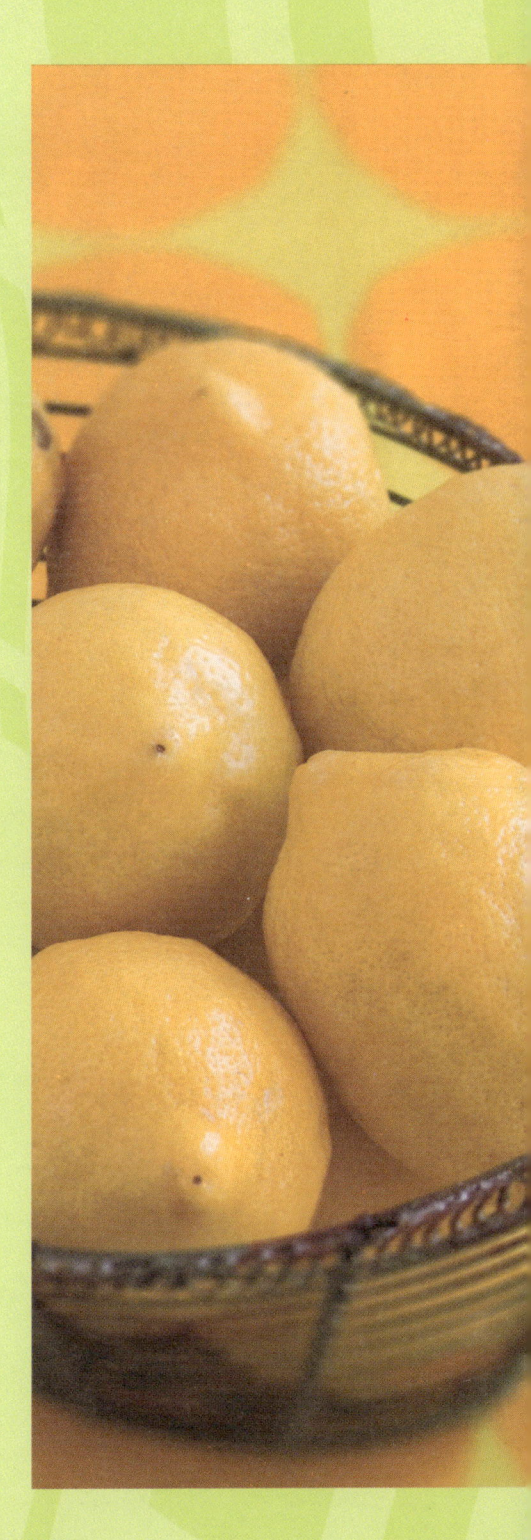

Juices

Fruit and vegetable juicing forms an integral chapter in naturopathic history. In Switzerland in the 1890s, well before the discovery of vitamins, Dr Max Bircher-Benner promoted the idea of eating raw food and drinking fruit and vegetable juices, proclaiming eating 'living' food could positively influence illness. In possibly the world's first holistic clinic, Life Force, Bircher-Benner incorporated exercise and psychotherapy (influenced by the work of Sigmund Freud) with juicing. In New York in the 1940s, Dr Max Gerson ran a successful sanatorium that centred around juicing and hydrotherapy, to treat cancer and other illnesses. Well before his time, Gerson promoted the health benefits of eating organically grown food.

Fruit and vegetable juices provide an easily digested and concentrated source of vitamins, minerals, enzymes and other phytonutrients.

But juicing should never replace eating the 'real thing'. For one, juicing loses valuable fibre; for another, we need to chew our food to maintain a healthy digestive tract.

If you're a novice juicer, start with a base juice of pear, carrot, orange or apple, and add from there. As a general rule of thumb, mix fruit with fruit and vegetable with vegetable, but there are some delicious exceptions, such as orange and carrot, and apple and celery. Be creative and playful and you'll soon find a repertoire of juices to suit your mood and wellbeing. If the juice tastes too strong, dilute it with water or increase the proportion of base juice.

Fruit and vegetables should be as fresh as possible and raw. The exceptions are frozen berries, which are often less expensive and available year-round. And it's fine to use stewed dried apricots where fresh apricots are unavailable. Organic fruit and vegetables are the best choice. If you're unable to buy organic produce, scrub the outside of fruit and vegetables to remove surface pesticides before juicing. Children love juices, too; for children under the age of 12, dilute juice with about one-third water.

JUICE	BENEFIT
Apple	Good all-round fruit for juicing, which is rich in vitamins, minerals and trace elements. Apples can relieve indigestion, constipation and, when diluted, diarrhoea. They also lower blood pressure and cholesterol.
Apricots	Rich in betacarotene, which the body converts to vitamin A, and iron, apricots are good for upset tummies, anaemia, cholesterol and skin problems. Soak dried apricots if fresh ones aren't available.

Beetroot Strong to taste (but surprisingly sweet), beetroot has a powerful effect on the body. Rich in minerals and antioxidants, it's a powerful blood tonic and cleanser. It's also valued as a digestive aid and liver stimulant, and is often used in alternative cancer treatments. Its strong red colour harmlessly colours stools and urine.

Cabbage Cabbage is well known for its antioxidant and detoxifying properties. It's also good for healing ulcers affecting the gastrointestinal tract, as well as liver problems and cancer prevention.

Carrot Carrot juice is the most popular vegetable juice because it tastes so delicious. A good source of betacarotene, carrot juice helps heal mucous membranes of the intestinal tract, bladder and lungs. Valuable for the heart, eyesight and circulation.

Celery A little bitter, with a pleasant savoury taste, celery is calming to the nervous system; it's also beneficial in reducing fluid retention. Good for gout, arthritis and rheumatism.

Cranberry Cranberries contain loads of vitamin C and antioxidants, and cranberry juice can help treat and prevent cystitis. Frozen cranberries can be used when fresh ones aren't available.

Cucumber Cucumber is a diuretic, so great for easing fluid retention. It also helps cool the body in fever and menopause, and helps regulate high blood pressure,

Grapefruit Excellent for liver and gall bladder conditions. It's also the classic weight-loss breakfast drink. Pink grapefruit contains lycopene, which is believed to lower the risk of prostate and other cancers. Grapefruit juice can interfere with some medications, so check with your GP before drinking it.

Lemon A good source of vitamin C and bioflavonoids, lemon juice is good for the skin, liver, constipation, veins and the immune system. A time-honoured recipe is to drink the juice of half a lemon in hot water with honey first thing in the morning. Squeezing lemon juice over food aids iron absorption.

Orange A reliable source of vitamin C, orange juice is a familiar favourite. Helpful for the immune system, colds and increasing iron absorption.

Parsley This herb is often included in vegetable juices thanks to its high mineral content, iron, calcium and potassium. It's also rich in vitamins A and C. A useful diuretic and anti-inflammatory.

Pear Pears are rich in soluble fibre, making them valuable as a bowel regulator. They're also good for lowering cholesterol. Pears are one of the least allergic foods.

Pineapple Pineapple contains bromelain, a protein-digesting enzyme that helps treat joint pain and inflammation. Pineapple juice helps digestion, relieves fluid retention, constipation and arthritis; it's also good for sore throats.

Rockmelon Delicious, cooling and refreshing, rockmelon contains antioxidants that help lower cholesterol.

Spinach A rich source of iron, magnesium and other minerals, spinach is good for anaemia, constipation and period problems.

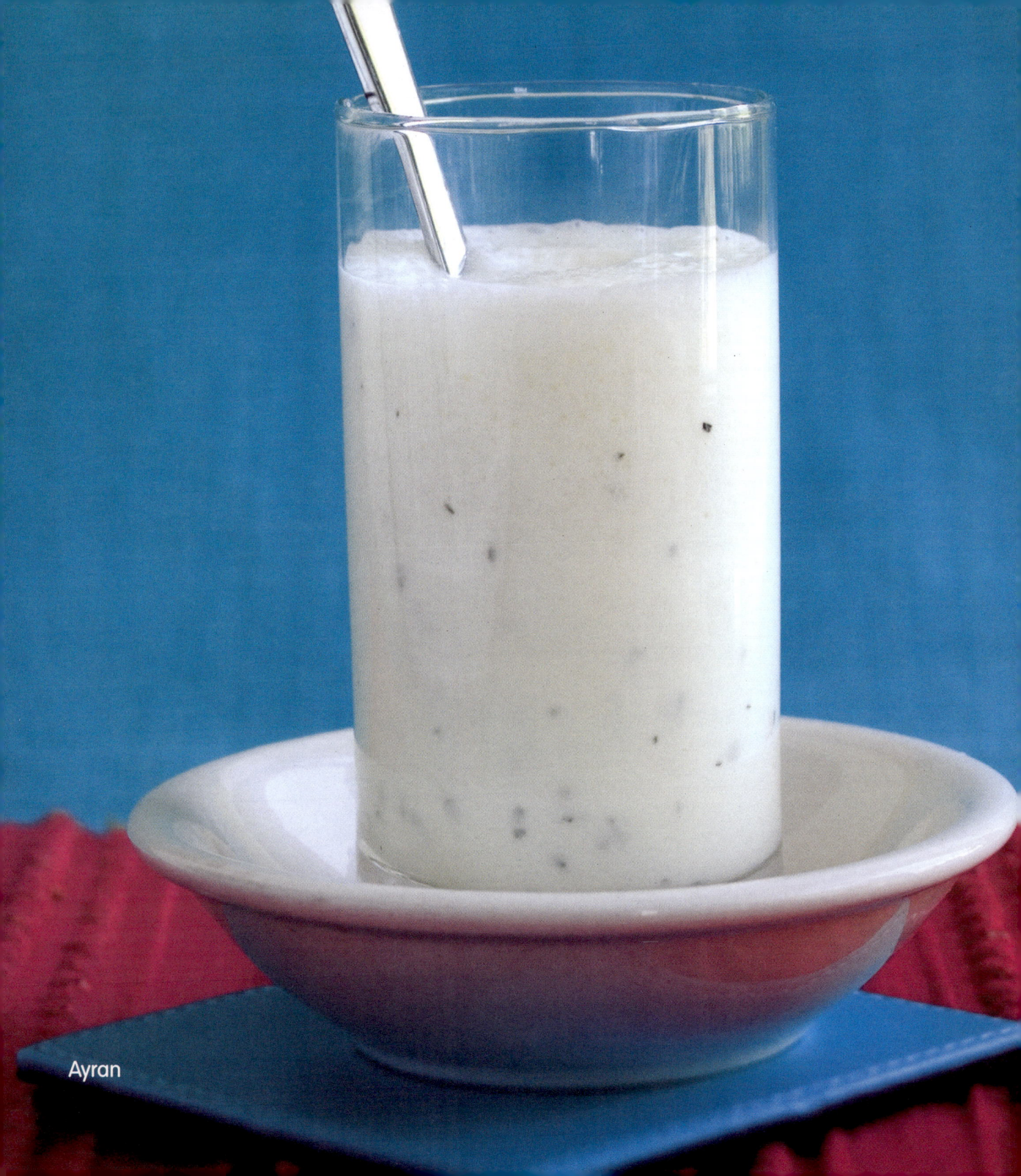

Ayran

Ginger

Ginger is both food and medicine. A traditional ingredient in cold, flu and digestive remedies, this versatile spice also warms cold fingers and toes. And it possesses anti-inflammatory powers, which makes it a popular arthritis remedy. Ginger is particularly effective in relieving nausea, from motion to morning sickness. It also eases tummy and bowel complaints, including diverticulitis pain. Additionally, ginger lowers blood cholesterol and reduces blood pressure.

Ginger can be used in a myriad of ways: in tea, in tablet form, crystallised, in compresses, and in the cooking of both sweet and savoury dishes. Ginger tea is just the thing for colds, flu, wind and nausea. Finely chop 2 centimetres of unpeeled fresh ginger root, place in a cup or teapot, pour over boiling water, leave for 3–5 minutes, and add a little honey or lemon to taste.

Ginger compresses, while fiddly, are fabulous for easing period cramps and muscle or joint pain. Grate a cupful of ginger into the middle of a cloth or tea towel, then fold to form a ginger parcel. Place in a shallow bowl and pour over 1 cup of boiling water. Leave until bearably hot. Gently squeeze and place on painful area, wrap body part and compress with plastic wrap. Wrap again in a towel, relax and keep warm for 20 minutes before unravelling.

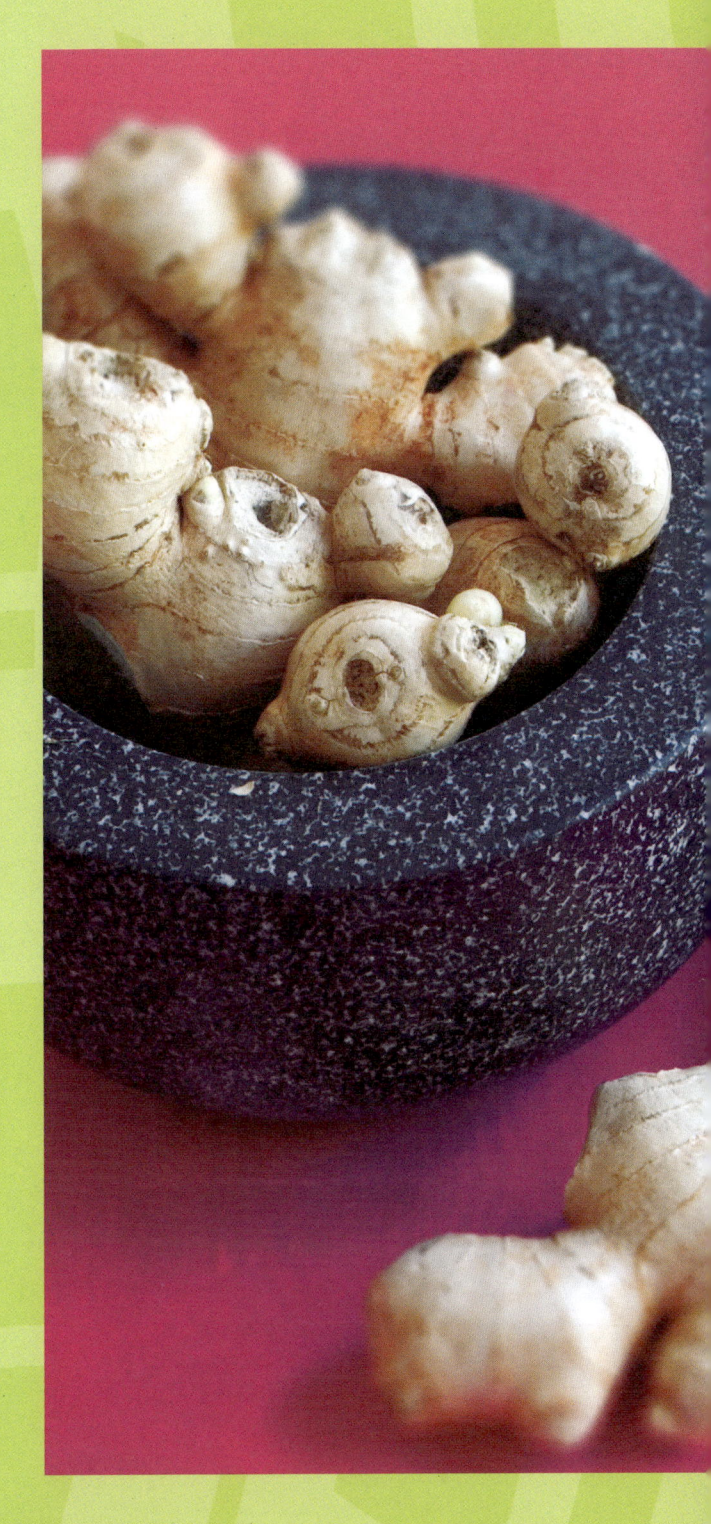

AYRAN

This is a delicious Turkish yoghurt drink that is perfect mid-morning or afternoon.

2 cups natural yoghurt
2 cups chilled water
2 teaspoons dried, crushed mint leaves
pinch of sea salt

Place yoghurt and water in a blender and whizz until mixture is smooth and frothy.

Add mint and salt.

Place ice cubes in 4 glasses and top with ayran.

SERVES 4

PEAR & GINGER JUICE

The best time to drink this juice is mid-afternoon when you need a sugar fix. It will give you a great boost.

8 ripe pears, washed and quartered
12cm/5in piece of ginger

Put pears and ginger in a juicer. Stir well.

Add a little cold water if ginger taste is too strong.

Place ice cubes in 4 glasses and top with pear and ginger juice.

SERVES 4

CARROT, APPLE & ORANGE JUICE

This is a particularly good combination of juices for when you're feeling under the weather.

8 carrots, washed and cut into halves
4 apples, washed and cut into quarters
4 oranges, peeled and cut into quarters

Process carrots, apples and oranges in a juicer, a piece at a time. Stir well.

Place ice cubes in 4 glasses and top with juice.

SERVES 4

PEPPERMINT TEA WITH GINGER

Peppermint is not only great for digestion, it is also excellent for easing tension.

1 tablespoon loose peppermint tea or 6 tea bags
½ cup mint leaves
2 tablespoons grated ginger
4 cups boiling water
1 tablespoon honey
12 mint leaves, extra

Place peppermint tea or tea bags, mint and ginger in a teapot and top with boiling water. Set aside to infuse for 15 minutes.

Strain tea into a jug, add honey and stir until dissolved.

Cool tea in the refrigerator for 2 hours.

Place ice cubes in 4 glasses, top with peppermint tea and 3 mint leaves.

SERVES 4

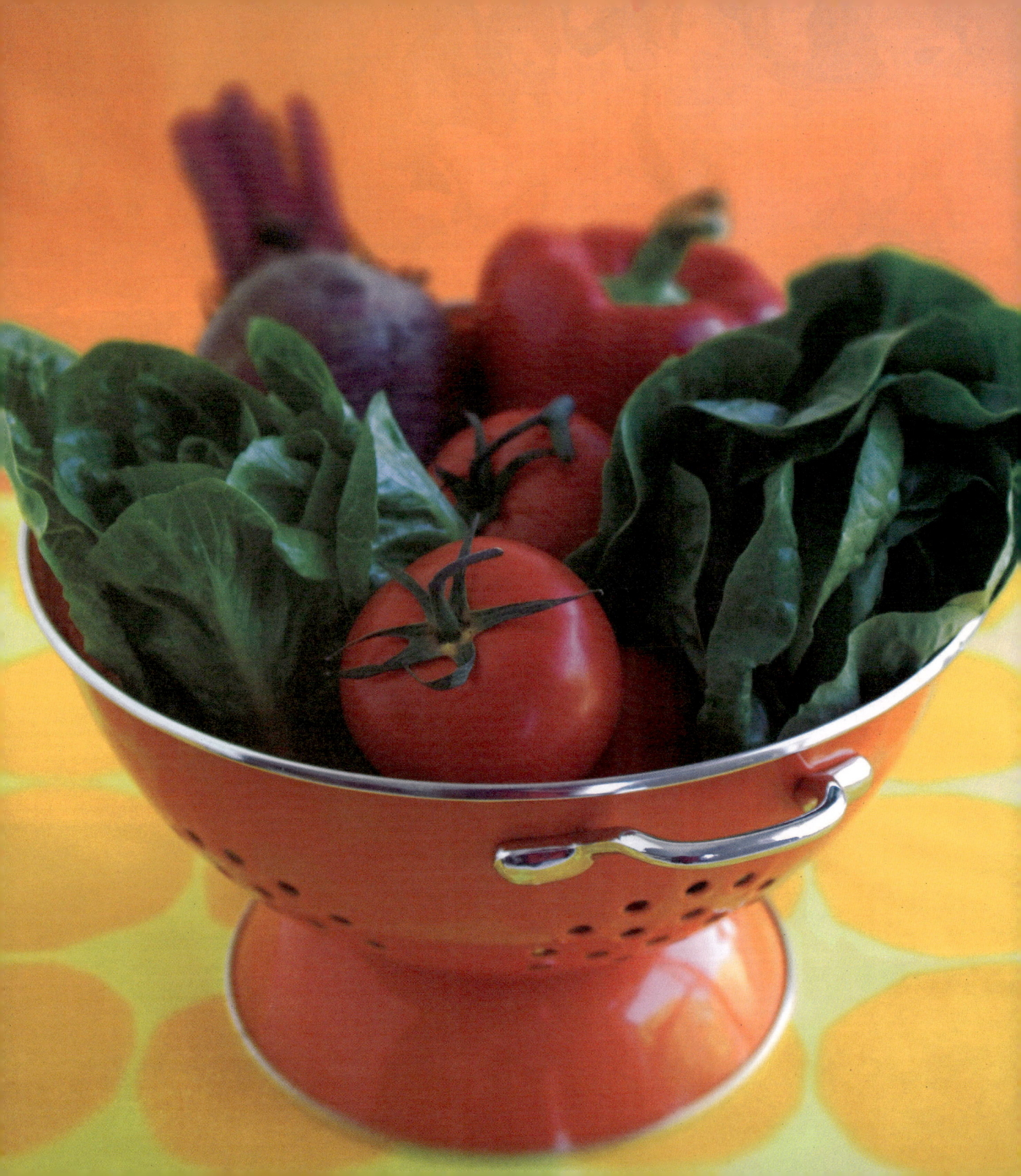

Antioxidants

Most fruit and vegetables contain antioxidants. Antioxidants prevent the damage caused by free radicals, thought to be partly responsible for diseases, such as heart disease, cancer, macular degeneration, arthritis, autoimmune conditions and many signs and symptoms of ageing, including wrinkles. The discovery of antioxidants and what they do in the body has transformed the old-fashioned message of eating fresh fruit and vegetables and whole grains into scientific good sense.

You may already be familiar with antioxidants such as vitamins A, C and E and minerals such as zinc and selenium. Fruits, vegetables, whole grains, legumes, nuts and seeds are all great sources of these micronutrients. In the last couple of decades, new compounds called phytonutrients have been found in plant foods that are also antioxidants—terrific news for the prevention and treatment of disease. For example, catechins, which are good for preventing heart disease and cancer, are found in green and black tea, red wine and cocoa; lycopene, which helps prevent prostate cancer, is found in cooked tomatoes and ruby grapefruit; curcumin, which is good for the liver, is found in the yellow Indian spice turmeric; indoles, which are both detoxifying and antioxidants, are found in abundance in broccoli and other vegetables in the Cruciferous family.

As a rule of thumb, the deeper the colour in the vegetable or fruit, the more phytonutrients and antioxidants. Many antioxidants are found in the skin and seeds of fruit and vegetables, so think twice before you peel. Also include a rainbow of coloured fruits and vegetables (orange, green and red) in your diet every day.

VEGETABLE COCKTAIL

This is a wonderful cocktail to have when you can't spare the time to sit down to lunch but need something to keep you going.

8 carrots, washed and cut into halves
1 bunch of celery, washed and cut into halves
4 beetroots, washed, scrubbed and cut into quarters
12cm/5in piece of ginger
4 lemons, peeled and quartered
1 bunch of parsley, washed
4 garlic cloves (optional)

Put all vegetables through a juicer, a little at a time. Stir well.

Place ice cubes in 4 glasses and top with the vegetable cocktail.

SERVES 4

SPICED TOMATO JUICE

This is a good drink for mid-morning, or to serve to teetotallers at drinks parties.

8 ice cubes
4 cups unsweetened tomato juice
juice of 1 lemon
1 tablespoon Worcestershire sauce
8 drops Tabasco
1 teaspoon celery salt
black pepper, to taste
4 lemon wedges

Place ice cubes in a large jug and top with tomato juice.

Add lemon juice, sauces, celery salt and pepper. Stir well.

Place a lemon wedge in each of 4 glasses and pour over tomato juice.

SERVES 4

Herbs

Fresh herbs not only add colour and flavour, they can transform a meal from merely nutritious to a positive health fest. Try experimenting with these in your juices and cooking.

Basil   Basil is good for the nervous system, helps digestion and relieves headaches and flatulence. Basil is also beneficial to acne sufferers and insomniacs.

Coriander   Providing a piquant flavour that lends itself to delicate dishes, coriander is also wonderful for digestion, including bloating and flatulence. It's also believed to enhance male potency.

Dill   Dill has been used historically to soothe colic in babies, and is also good for adult digestive difficulties including bloating, nausea and flatulence.

Mint   Mint is used medicinally for all sorts of conditions, including heartburn, nausea, stomach ache, diverticulitis, colds and flu.

Oregano   Another herb to aid digestion, oregano is also used for respiratory problems, including bronchitis, coughs and even asthma.

Parsley   A good source of vitamins A and C and iron, parsley also contains phytohormones, making it a fine herb for menopause. Parsley is also used for kidney and bladder problems, including fluid retention.

Thyme   An antiseptic herb, thyme is effective against bacteria and fungi. It is excellent for the respiratory and digestive systems and is used herbally for conditions as diverse as sinusitis, candida, coughs, urinary tract infections and flatulence.

> **Fresh herbs are preferable to dried as they contain more essential oils and vitamins, but it's better to have dried herbs than none at all.**

feelgood food

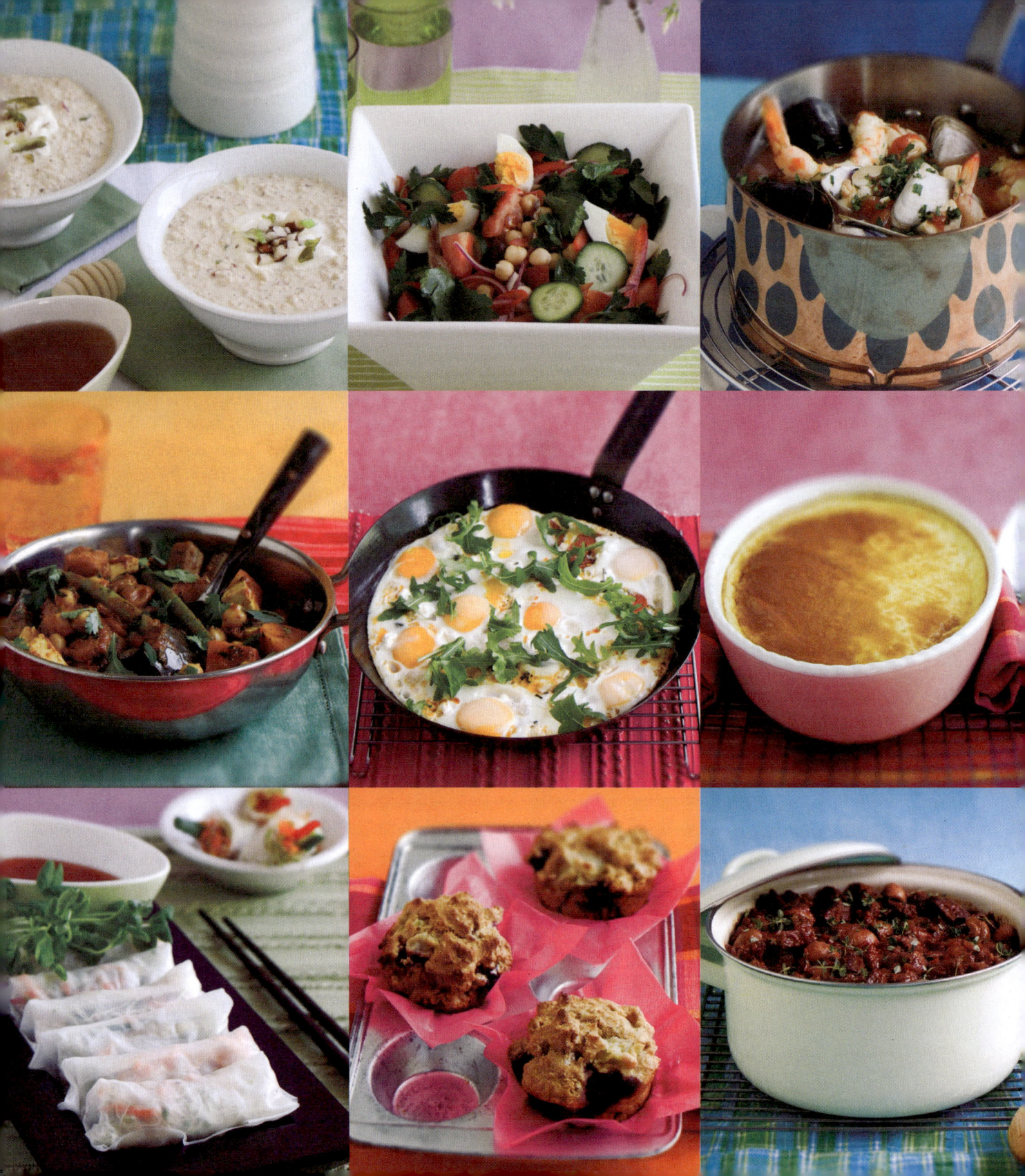

Menu plans

The following menu plans will help you create meals for a day or a week that are nutritionally balanced and delicious too.

By including recipes that contain foods that help prevent or treat various conditions, you know you are doing the best possible thing for yourself and your family.

The following are suggested menu plans for 2 weeks based on the recipes in this book.

Week 1

	Breakfast	Snack	Lunch	Snack	Dinner
Day 1	Protein shake	Pumpkin & pepita Muffins	Mediterranean salad	fresh fruit	Roast lamb with root vegetables
Day 2	Baked brown rice pudding with apricots	Olive paste with crackers or crispbread	Omelette with feta & dill	Ayran	Lentil stew
Day 3	Porridge	Chickpea & tahini dip	Brown rice & tuna salad	Fresh fruit	Flathead fillets with potato & herb salad
Day 4	Mango, banana & tofu smoothie	Oat & sunflower-seed cookies	Tuna salad	Pear & ginger juice	Honey & soy chicken
Day 5	Poached eggs with spinach & yoghurt	Rice paper rolls	Carrot & ginger soup with coriander	Fresh fruit	Almost shepherd's pie
Day 6	Protein shake	Beetroot & yoghurt dip	Beef salad	Vegetable cocktail	Penne with tuna, olives & capers Poached pears with chocolate sauce
Day 7	Scrambled eggs with basil	Chocolate & raspberry muffins	Red lentil soup	Fresh fruit	Moroccan lamb Pumpkin pudding

Week 2

	Breakfast	Snack	Lunch	Snack	Dinner
Day 1	Bircher muesli	Spicy avocado mash on garlic toast	Zucchini slice	Fresh fruit	Roast beef with mustard, chives & garlic
Day 2	Protein shake	Pumpkin & pepita muffins	Mediterranean salad	Carrot, apple & orange juice	Spaghetti with chicken, cherry tomatoes, basil & pine nuts
Day 3	Toasted English muffin with cottage cheese, tomato & avocado	Beetroot & yoghurt dip	Steak sandwich with horseradish cream & snow pea sprouts	Hot cocoa	Chickpea curry
Day 4	Fruit salad with mint & yoghurt	Olive paste	Tuna salad	Fresh fruit	Lamb cutlets with mashed potato, garlic green beans & roast tomato
Day 5	Toasted muesli with yoghurt	Eggplant & tahini dip	Lentil salad	Spiced tomato juice	Marlin with green beans, pesto & roast tomatoes
Day 6	Sardines & tomato on toast	Oat & sunflower-seed cookies	Spanish omelette	Fresh fruit	Chilli con carne with avocado & yoghurt topping Ricotta cheesecake
Day 7	Eggs with tomato, feta & herbs	Apple & blueberry muffins	Pea soup	Pear & ginger juice	Braised beef with mushrooms, red wine & herbs Apple & blackberry crumble

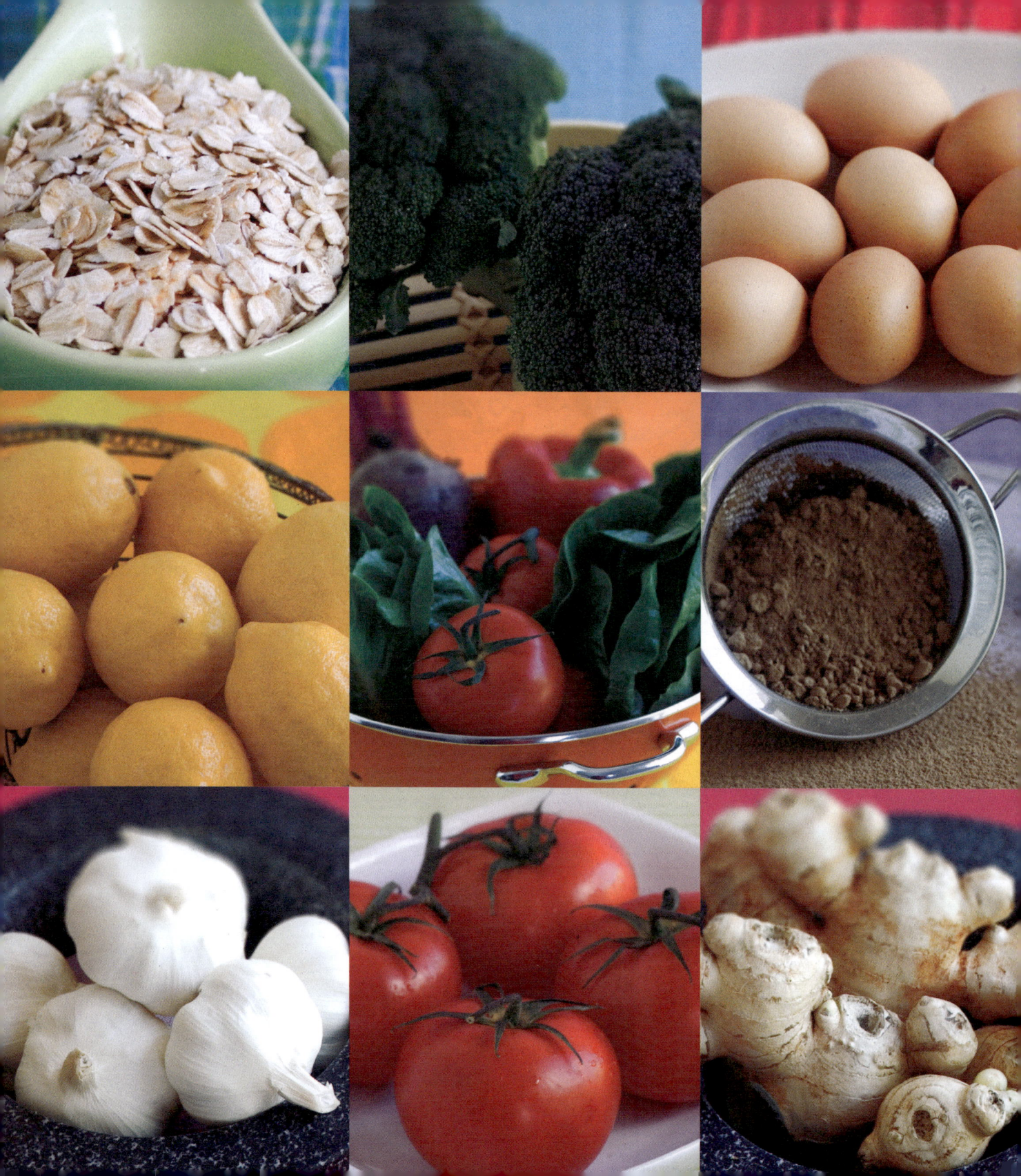

Your pantry

The following list of all the ingredients used throughout the book will be a godsend when shopping.

CANNED FISH, VEGETABLES & FRUIT
Anchovy fillets
Apricots in natural juice
Cannellini beans
Capers
Chickpeas
Diced pie apples
Diced tomatoes
Kalamata olives
Kalamata olives, pitted
Pimento-stuffed green olives
Red kidney beans
Sardines
Tuna

CEREALS & BREADS
Bread
Cornflakes
English muffins
Fruit bread
Rolled oats

DAIRY & DAIRY SUBSTITUTES
Butter
Coconut milk
Cottage cheese
Cream
Eggs
Feta
Milk
Natural yoghurt
Parmesan
Protein powder
Fresh ricotta
Tofu—silken and firm

DRIED FRUIT, NUTS & SEEDS
Almonds (natural, slivered and flaked)
Apricots
Cashews, roasted unsalted
Coconut, shredded
LSA (linseeds, sunflower seeds and almonds)
Peanuts, roasted unsalted
Pepitas
Pine nuts
Sesame seeds
Sultanas
Sunflower seeds
Tahini, hulled
Walnuts

FLOURS & OTHER BAKING INGREDIENTS
Cocoa
Baking powder
Brown rice flour
Buckwheat flour
Dark choc bits
Dark cooking chocolate
Filo pastry
Fine polenta
Molasses
Plain flour
Wholemeal flour

FRESH FISH, CHICKEN & MEAT
Beef mince
Chicken tenderloins
Chicken thigh fillets
Diced beef
Diced lamb
Fillet of beef
Fish fillets
Fish heads
Flathead fillets
Green prawns
Lamb cutlets
Marlin steaks
Mussels
Pippies or clams
Rump steak
Shoulder of lamb
Veal shanks

FRESH FRUIT
Apples
Avocados
Bananas
Berries
Cherry tomatoes
Kiwi fruit
Lemons
Limes
Mangoes
Oranges
Passionfruit
Pears
Roma tomatoes

FRESH HERBS
Baby rocket
Baby spinach
Basil
Broccoli sprouts
Chillies
Coriander
Dill
Ginger
Lemongrass
Mint
Oregano
Parsley
Rosemary
Salad sprouts
Snow pea sprouts
Thyme

FRESH VEGETABLES
Beetroot
Broccoli
Button mushrooms
Cabbage
Capsicum—red and green
Carrots
Celery
Cos lettuce
Eggplant
Garlic
Green beans

Lebanese cucumber
Okra
Onions
Potatoes
Pumpkin
Red cabbage
Snow peas
Spanish onions
Spinach
Spring onions
Sweet potato
Zucchini

FROZEN FRUIT & VEGETABLES

Blackberries
Blueberries
Mango cheeks
Mixed berries
Peas
Raspberries

HERBS & SPICES

Bay leaves
Cardamom, ground
Celery salt
Cinnamon, ground
Cinnamon, sticks
Chilli, ground
Cloves, whole
Cumin, ground
Harissa
Mint, crushed leaves
Mixed herbs, leaves
Nutmeg, ground
Paprika
Saffron
Turmeric, ground
Vanilla extract

JUICES, TEAS & OTHER DRINKS

Apple juice
Blackcurrant juice
Cocoa powder
Green tea
Orange juice
Peppermint tea
Red wine
Tomato juice
Soda water
White wine

OILS, COOKING SAUCES & CONDIMENTS

Black and white pepper
Chilli paste
Gelatine
Horseradish cream
Miso paste
Olive oil
Peppercorns
Rogan josh curry paste

Sea salt
Sesame oil
Soy sauce
Tabasco sauce
Tomato paste
Tomato purée
White wine vinegar
Wholegrain French mustard
Worcestershire sauce

PASTA, RICE & PULSES
Brown rice
Couscous
Dried lentils, red
Dried lentils, brown or green
Great northern beans, dried
Green split peas, dried
Penne
Rice paper sheets
Thin spaghetti

SWEETENERS
Brown sugar
Honey

Detox...
if you must

Detoxing has become as fashionable as Manolo Blahnik stilettoes. In certain circumstances a gentle detox is justified. But I have several 'problems' with the detox concept.

My first concern is that the average person's organs of detoxification and elimination (namely the liver, bowel, lungs, skin and kidneys) are already doing a perfectly adequate job. Day in, day out, these organs happily go about their business, in the most part willingly and without complaint. Imagine their shock when, one morning, they wake up to find themselves purged, rinsed and starved. In general, the body prefers status quo. It likes regular eating, sleeping and exercise patterns. Many detox programs are entered into after a period of partying or eating badly. While the intentions may be good, going directly from 'very bad' to 'very good' is in itself stressful. It's much better to err slightly and slowly get back on a healthy balanced track than to seesaw between two extremes.

My second concern is rather more esoteric. The word 'detoxification' implies we are toxic, which ties in with feelings of guilt and a cult of perfectionism. Going on a detox for some people is the equivalent of wearing a hair shirt, only more visible.

My last concern is far more cynical, (and I need to own up to personal 'stuff' as a former anorexic and exercise junkie). I believe that some people go on a detox to lose weight rapidly, pretending it's in the name of health. In the same way gym addicts pound their bodies to get into shape, it's more for vanity not health reasons. There's nothing wrong with trying to look your best, but both these things become obsessions.

Now that's off my chest, I feel much better. Perhaps it's better to view detox as a kick-start to a long-term healthier way of eating. Your detox could be a time to start or further other healthy habits such as exercise and meditation. Here is a gentle two-week detox plan to ease yourself in and out of.

> PLEASE CHECK WITH YOUR HEALTH-CARE PRACTITIONER TO DISCUSS WHETHER THIS KIND OF DETOX IS FOR YOU
>
> DETOXING IS NOT RECOMMENDED IF YOU'RE UNDER THE AGE OF 18, PREGNANT, UNDERWEIGHT OR SERIOUSLY ILL

WHAT TO ENJOY

All fruit, vegetables—preferably organic.
Legumes (eg, lentils, chickpeas, tofu and tempeh)
Fish (best eaten fresh, or canned in olive oil or spring water)
Raw nuts and seeds
Brown rice
Miso soup
Herbal teas

WHAT TO AVOID (THROUGHOUT THE DETOX)

Sugar
White flour products
Tea and coffee
Caffeine
Alcohol
Red meat
Deli meats
Fried food (stir-frying in olive oil is okay)

DAYS 1–14

- Start each day with the juice of half a lemon in hot water (honey optional).
- One juice daily—mixture of carrot, beetroot, celery and ginger.
- Drink 2 litres of water daily
- Drink one to two cups of detox tea (either Detox from Perfect Potion, or Glow from Tea Centre)
- Food is best eaten raw, lightly steamed, stir-fried or dry baked.

DAYS 3–12

This is the central core of the detox. In addition to the above, avoid the following foods:
Wheat
Milk products (except good quality natural yoghurt)
Chicken
Dried fruit
White rice

THINGS TO WATCH OUT FOR

Headaches—a throbbing headache is a common side effect of detoxing. Headaches often result when we remove caffeine and sugar from our diet. Usually, headaches appear 48 hours after starting the detox and should only last a day or so. However, some people may experience them for up to one week. The best thing to do is to drink plenty of water, and if you really can't stand it any longer, then take a Panadol.

Irritability—no one said detoxing was going to be fun. However, like the headaches, feeling 'blah' should only last a couple of days before you start to feel fantastic.

Constipation—for some people, a radical change in diet can cause their bowels to go on strike. Ease them back on track by adding two teaspoons of psyllium husks (or Metamucil) to a glass of water each day.

Your Food Journal

Just so you know exactly what you're putting in your mouth each day, how much you're exercising and how you're feeling, you might like to keep a food diary (see our sample diary opposite). We've left the following pages blank for you to get started.

sample diary for a day

6:00	cup of hot water with lemon juice; glass of water with a dash of apple juice
7:00	
8:00	glass of water; mug of soy milk coffee; protein shake with soy milk, strawberries, pear & banana
9:00	glass of water
10:00	glass of water; peach
11:00	vegetable cocktail
Noon	handful of raw almonds; glass of water
Comments	8km run at 6:30, good energy levels throughout morning.
1:00	glass of water
2:00	glass of water; tuna salad with lettuce, tomato, onion, carrot, cucumber, avocado, snow peas, capsicum, feta, oil & vinegar
3:00	glass of water
4:00	1 apple and blueberry muffin
5:00	cup of black tea
Comments	Feeling a little tired, looking forward to sitting down and having a glass of wine in front of TV
6:00	
7:00	glass of pinot noir; 1 rice paper roll
8:00	chilli con carne with avocado & yoghurt topping & corn chips; glass of pinot noir
9:00	2 pieces of dark chocolate
10:00	glass of water
Comments	Bed at 10:30

feelgood food

DAY 1		DAY 2	
6:00	_____	6:00	_____
7:00	_____	7:00	_____
8:00	_____	8:00	_____
9:00	_____	9:00	_____
10:00	_____	10:00	_____
11:00	_____	11:00	_____
Noon	_____	Noon	_____
Comments	_____	Comments	_____
1:00	_____	1:00	_____
2:00	_____	2:00	_____
3:00	_____	3:00	_____
4:00	_____	4:00	_____
5:00	_____	5:00	_____
Comments	_____	Comments	_____
6:00	_____	6:00	_____
7:00	_____	7:00	_____
8:00	_____	8:00	_____
9:00	_____	9:00	_____
10:00	_____	10:00	_____
Comments	_____	Comments	_____

DAY 3

6:00 _____
7:00 _____
8:00 _____
9:00 _____
10:00 _____
11:00 _____
Noon _____
Comments _____
1:00 _____
2:00 _____
3:00 _____
4:00 _____
5:00 _____
Comments _____
6:00 _____
7:00 _____
8:00 _____
9:00 _____
10:00 _____
Comments _____

DAY 4

6:00 _____
7:00 _____
8:00 _____
9:00 _____
10:00 _____
11:00 _____
Noon _____
Comments _____
1:00 _____
2:00 _____
3:00 _____
4:00 _____
5:00 _____
Comments _____
6:00 _____
7:00 _____
8:00 _____
9:00 _____
10:00 _____
Comments _____

feelgood food

Sensible eating diary

Name:

Condition:

What to eat:

What to avoid:

Sensible eating diary

Name: _____

Condition: _____
_____
_____

What to eat: _____
_____
_____
_____
_____
_____

What to avoid: _____
_____
_____
_____
_____
_____

Sensible eating diary

Name: _____

Condition: _____
_____
_____

What to eat: _____
_____
_____
_____
_____
_____
_____

What to avoid: _____
_____
_____
_____
_____
_____
_____

Sensible eating diary

Name: _____

Condition: _____
_____
_____

What to eat: _____
_____
_____
_____
_____
_____

What to avoid: _____
_____
_____
_____
_____
_____
_____

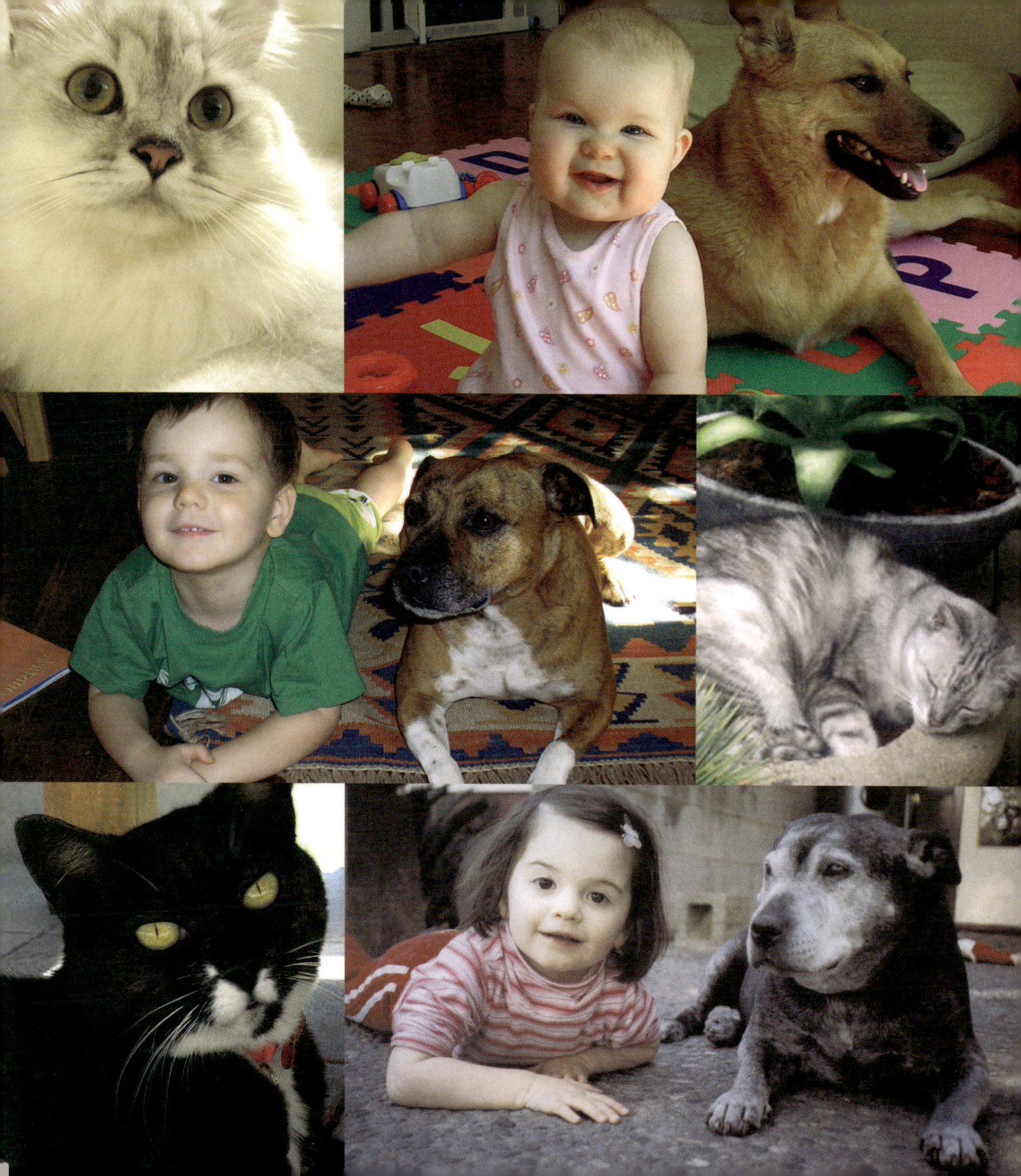

Don't forget the other members of your family

If you are a fan of natural medicine, there is no reason why your pooch or puss can't enjoy natural health too.

Just as vegetables are an important part of your diet, they should be part of your pet's too. The following is a favourite with canines, but your cat might be more fussy. Steam or microwave a mixture of carrot, pumpkin, broccoli and potato. Mash together. Mix a palm-size portion into your pet's meal of meat or biscuits each night. These vegetable portions freeze well. Give your pet roo meat, which is lean and full of iron and protein and is low in fat.

To improve your cat's or dog's immunity, give them a daily capsule of cod-liver oil for 1 month. If your animal detests capsules, and you detest being clawed and mauled, squeeze the contents of the capsule over their food. Adding crushed garlic (or a garlic oil capsule) to their food is another way to improve immunity.

There is no simpler way to rid yourself of friends than to have a lounge room that's a fleapit. Wash the dog and his blanky in wool wash (the one with eucalyptus oil added), rinse in cold water, then towel dry the dog, and tumble dry the blanky. Fleas and Dracula have at least one thing in common: they both hate garlic, so carry out the garlic treatment mentioned above.

Is your pet's fur dull and listless? Swap their beef or chicken for a can of omega-3-rich tuna, salmon or sardines. Flaxseed oil is also excellent for unsightly fur, as well as dry skin and eczema. Add a dessertspoonful to their meal. To make your animal even more glamorous, add $1/4$–$1/2$ teaspoon of brewer's yeast to their food.

ACKNOWLEDGEMENTS

Gül McCarty

The concept of *Feelgood Food* was the result of my passion for good food and good health, and I asked Mim Beim if she would join me in writing a book on the topic. Mim's vast knowledge of naturopathy and nutrition, delivered in an entertaining style, is always so easy to understand and an absolute joy to read. I'd like to thank Mim for agreeing to co-write this book and for guiding me through the journey. I treasure her friendship. Thanks to my beautiful nephew, Nick McHugh, for being the catalyst; Jo Mackay for liking the concept and running with it; Helen Littleton for her incredible positive energy; my family for giving me their unconditional love; Milly, my cat, for staying by my side; and my loving husband, Ross, for being my soul mate and always giving me the support I need. This book is dedicated to Rocky.

Mim Beim

When Gül McCarty first approached me with the concept of *Feelgood Food* I was struck by her passionate desire for people to eat well, and feel the benefits. A woman who walks her talk, Gül is testament to the benefits of a healthy lifestyle, and delicious food! Thanks to Jo Mackay who took us up on the idea; the fabulous Stuart Neal who said yes; Helen Littleton, a woman of action; and of course my darling Bill. This book is dedicated to Greg Ockenden (about time!)

The information in this book should not be substituted for the advice obtained from consultation with, and treatment by, your health practitioner. Nor is it intended to directly or indirectly prescribe the use of various remedies without the consent of your health practitioner. If you are under medical care for any condition, seek the advice of your health practitioner before acting on any suggestions in this book, and do not make any adjustments to prescribed medication or treatment regime without their prior approval.

Published by ABC Books for the
AUSTRALIAN BROADCASTING CORPORATION
GPO Box 9994 Sydney NSW 2001

Copyright © Mim Beim & Gül McCarty 2006

First published May 2006

All rights reserved. No part of this publication may be reproduced, stored in a retrieval system or transmitted in any form or by any means, electronic, mechanical, photocopying, recording or otherwise, without the prior written permission of the Australian Broadcasting Corporation.

Beim, Mim, 1960- .
Feelgood food: recipes & menus for healthier Australian families.

ISBN 0 7333 1602 6.

1. Cookery (Natural foods). 2. Diet therapy - Australia.
3. Family - Health and hygiene - Australia. I. McCarty, Gul.
II. Australian Broadcasting Corporation. III. Title.

641.563

Designed by saso content & design pty ltd
Typeset in Swiss 721 11pt by saso content & design
Colour reproduction by Graphic Print Group, Adelaide
Printed in Hong Kong China, by Quality Printing

5 4 3 2 1

Key: t=top, m=middle, b=bottom, l=left, r=right
Additional photography: Digitalvision/Lorry Eason Freshly Grown: p50 tl, tm, bm, br; p70 ml, mr; p91 t, m; p115 t, b; p138 tm, bl, br; p156 tm, ml, mr, bm; p169 t, m, b; p70 tm, ml, bm.
Istock p67 b; p79; p119 t,b.